Nino's Epiphanies

A Chiropractor Explains to You
and Your Doctor What Really Causes
and Cures Back and Joint Pain

Dr. John A. Ramsey

Nino's Epiphanies

Contents

Acknowledgements

I want to thank and extend my deepest appreciation to several people who made this book possible: I thank my son, Keith Ippolito, for his support and encouragement, as well as for helping me fashion my many discoveries, memories, and accumulated knowledge into a manuscript. I next wish to thank my editor, Lee Sakellarides, who put to use not only her superb command of the English language and writing skills in editing the manuscript, but also her considerable and invaluable publishing industry savvy in the process of turning it literally into a book. For legal advice in the publication of this book, my thanks to Baker & Daniels and attorney Kevin R. Erdman. Thanks also to my friend Julia Herring for her faith in me and willingness to take advantage of my knowledge and techniques in overcoming more than a few health problems over the last few years, sometimes in ways that surprised us both. Finally, I want to give thanks for having been blessed with the opportunity to treat the many thousands of patients who walked into my office over the years, as without them I would have had no epiphanies and there would be no book to write.

CHAPTER 1
"Nino! Where Did You Come From?"

One day a woman brought her sixteen-year-old daughter into my office and asked if I could help her. I'll never forget the sight of this girl walking into my office encased in a plaster body cast that extended from her chest to her pelvis. She had suffered since birth from thoracic scoliosis and had, up to that time, been under the care of an orthopedist. Before I took her history, I had her mother remove the cast, revealing her abnormally protruding right shoulder blade. She was underweight, malnourished, and had not yet started to menstruate. She was also depressed, nervous, unable to sleep, and suffered from persistent headaches and back pain. If I recall correctly, she was not then attending school.

Not surprisingly, upon examining her in a standing position, I found taut spinal muscles, taut pelvic muscles, cervical muscle contraction, and pain in her thighs and legs. Though I don't know how or why she and her mother ended up in my office, and I hadn't treated a patient with scoliosis before, I told them I would do my best to help

Nutritionally, I placed her on a diet that included six eight-ounce glasses of distilled water a day.

Musculoskeletally, I immediately began reversal massage on her problem areas, and some of her pain subsided before she left my office on the very first visit. I set her next, and subsequent, appointments three days apart, and instructed her to rest in bed in the meantime.

When she came back for the second visit, she walked into my office without the plaster body cast. She was feeling better, was less nervous, and had less pain.

One month later she was free of pain, sleeping better, and was even able to get to my office by herself, since her mother was unable to bring her.

Two months later she had her first period and was apparently feeling much better. Shortly afterwards she stopped coming for treatment and I lost contact with her. To my knowledge, though, she never wore a cast after that first visit.

Several years later, she paid me a surprise visit—to show me her baby. I can't remember exactly what we discussed, but I couldn't help but interpret her visit to me with her child as her way of thanking me for helping to make it possible for her to live a more normal life.

* * * * * * *

My mother, Mary, often said to me, "Nino! Where did you come from?" but never got an answer. Her question was only half rhetorical. She never denied that she and my father, Louis Ippolito, were my biological parents, and she had no doubt where they had come from—Regalbuto, Sicily. Still, my mother clearly felt that, somehow—perhaps in a more spiritual sense—I was not really hers, that sometime between my conception and delivery I had taken an out-of-this-world diversion during which something had tampered with my persona. She just couldn't believe she had conceived someone like me! I couldn't blame her for feeling that way. At an early age I manifested the same unconventionality I do today. While my sisters and the rest of the kids in the neighborhood played with dolls and toys, I spent my childhood alone taking things apart to see what made them work.

I received my draft notice in February 1944. My induction eligibility physical indicated that I had an ulcer, but I didn't believe it. I asked them if they would accept me if I could prove that I didn't, and they said they would. That May, after a private medical physical proved I didn't have an ulcer, I was permitted to enlist in the Army Air Force Aviation Cadets. Unfortunately, testing revealed that I had a depth perception problem, permanently grounding my dream of becoming a fighter pilot. I was then assigned to and completed the radio, radar, and advanced radar schools, and eventually became a GCA (Ground Control Approach) equipment maintenance instructor. This equipment was used to help land airplanes during nighttime or zero-ceiling weather. I remained in this position until I was honorably discharged in May 1946.

As was the case with many of my fellow ex-servicemen, the G.I. Bill was available to finance the college education I desired. My high school chemistry teacher had written in my yearbook that I would one day be a famous chemist. Influenced by my love of chemistry and the fact that my uncle was a pharmacist, I decided to become a pharmacist, too. As thousands of other discharged soldiers and I were flooding all the professional colleges, and the admissions office at the College of Pharmacy at State University of New York in Buffalo had a long waiting list, my sisters helped me apply to a number of other pharmacy colleges. Eventually I was accepted by the University of Oklahoma Pharmacy School. As the fall semester would not begin for several months, my sister helped me get a job at Linde Aire Lab, designing and making experimental glass research equipment.

One day when I returned home from work, I saw my father and grandfather working in a deep pit repairing a water pipe leak. As I attempted to help my father out of the pit by pulling on his arm, I injured his shoulder. My father asked me to drive him to see a chiropractor—a health care profession which was alien to me.

The chiropractor, who, to my surprise, was blind, led us to the treatment room and told my father to lie face down on the treatment table. At the end of the treatment, to which I paid little attention, my father felt better. The chiropractor then turned to me and asked me if I'd been recently discharged from the military, and I told him that I had. He then asked what my plans were. I told him that I was enrolled in a pharmacy college. He said that was fine, and then asked if I would be interested in a chiropractic career, adding that there was no competition in that field. This instantly caught my attention and stirred my interest, as it reminded me that thousands of my fellow ex-GI's were flooding every professional school in the country. I told him that, prior to my father's visit to his office, not only was I unacquainted with chiropractic, I wasn't even aware that chiropractic existed.

He explained that chiropractic diagnosis and treatment are based on the principle that when a slipped vertebra pinches a nerve, it prevents that nerve from sending energy to a specific part of the body. As a result, that body part, deprived of that nerve energy, will weaken and become sick and painful. He said that the chiropractor uses no drugs, but rather uses spinal manipulation to release this pinched nerve, thereby restoring the flow of energy to the sick body part. I was fascinated with his description of the natural aspects of chiropractic healing. I told the doctor I would give some thought to a career as a chiropractor, and he suggested I look into attending his alma mater, Lincoln Chiropractic College, in Indianapolis, Indiana.

Reflecting on my conversation with the chiropractor, I decided to get a "second opinion" on the merits of a career in chiropractic. I asked our family doctor what he thought. Without giving specific reasons, he strongly advised against my becoming a chiropractor. Faced with these conflicting opinions, I let the matter simmer in my subconscious until one day when I strolled into the glass blowers' area at work and received the inspiration I needed to end the tug-of-war.

Several of the employees were discussing their experiences with chiropractic. One mentioned he was relieved of headaches, while another praised the healing of his acute low backache. I suddenly experienced a flashback to when I was nine years old. I had just finished supper, and was walking into the yard when, for no apparent reason, I vomited a bright red substance. My mother called the doctor, who, without examining me or questioning me about pain or any other symptoms, diagnosed acute appendicitis, and ordered an immediate appendectomy. Several weeks later, I recalled that I had eaten sugar beets at supper that evening, which explained the blood-like color of my stomach contents.

The memory of having undergone needless surgery due to a hasty misdiagnosis—by the same doctor who advised me against attending chiropractic school—convinced me to ignore his advice and take the chiropractor's. I applied to and was accepted at Lincoln Chiropractic School for the fall semester of 1946, and enrolled in an accelerated program which would allow me to finish the four-year course in three years. I moved to Indianapolis, began attending classes at Lincoln, and found a part-time job to supplement the $65 a month, plus tuition and books, I received under the GI Bill.

CHAPTER 2
Blinkin' At Lincoln

When I opened my practice in Buffalo in 1950, chiropractic was still in its infancy. New York, as with all but a few other states, had no licensing requirements for practitioners of chiropractic. And as far as I could tell, there were only a few other chiropractors in Buffalo.

Chiropractic was, at that time, alien not only to my family and friends, but to the public. It suddenly dawned on me how difficult it was going to be to market chiropractic as a concept, let alone my practice. Thus, for financial reasons, I was obliged to support my family by working 40 hours a week as a technical writer at Sylvania Electronics.

In addition to these challenges, I encountered in my practice in Buffalo a more formidable problem—lack of results. Suffice it to say that, in my application of what I learned at Lincoln, I wasn't getting the results with patients that they needed to thrive and I needed to survive. It would be helpful for you to understand what I was taught at Lincoln so you can appreciate how I strove to overcome numerous obstacles to success by embarking on a journey that was and is filled with astonishing experiences and revelations about the nature of the human body—experiences that led to the epiphanies that ultimately formed my philosophy and approach to healing.

As I recall, Lincoln Chiropractic College was started by two or three successful chiropractors (who drove around in Cadillacs to prove it) and a radiologist. Their goal was to make the school the flagship institution of chiropractic education; to make sure that, through its faculty and curriculum, its graduates had the best possible training in the sciences and the finest clinical skills. I remember talking with these founding fathers, who, though accessible and visible, never taught any classes.

During my first year at Lincoln, I learned there were three different chiropractic "schools of thought," each named for its own method: Palmer, Logan, and Lincoln. At a school based on the Palmer principles, pain and sickness were caused by slippage of the atlas and axis vertebrae located on top of the neck and at the base of the skull. A Logan school taught that the sacrum, which is located immediately below the last lumbar vertebra, is the primary origination point of disease. At Lincoln, the belief was that ill health was caused by slippage of any of the spinal vertebrae, whether atlas, axis, or sacrum. Several years would pass before I would understand what these different chiropractic schools of thought really said about the validity of chiropractic theory, not to mention the future of chiropractic itself—and my own future as a chiropractor.

I often wondered about these widely divergent philosophies, though I did not see their theoretical differences as particularly revolutionary. In fact, I questioned the validity of all three. But I dismissed my misgivings for several reasons. First, how could I, a freshman, credibly challenge something about which I then knew nothing? Besides, medical doctors often treated the same illness with different approaches, so, logically, why couldn't chiropractic, too?

Second, as a busy student I simply didn't have the time or mental energy to question anything. Lincoln students had two choices: stay and demonstrate our utmost faith in Lincoln chiropractic, or leave. If we stayed, we had but one objective: to graduate!

The third and most important reason arose from the fragile, often-attacked legitimacy of chiropractic in the healthcare field. To the medical community, which refused to validate any of the three theories, chiropractic was anathema. They called us "the occult." As the years went by chiropractic would have to fight in court in a number of states for its right to exist as a profession—a fight it would win. At that time, though, with the medical community ever ready to pounce on an opportunity to eradicate chiropractic, Lincoln students were required to maintain a choirboy image. We had to dress in shirts and ties, and our behavior had to be exemplary. We were told that any conduct on or off campus that in any way reflected negatively on Lincoln would result in expulsion. Given the paramount importance of graduation, I kept my nose clean and my thoughts to myself.

Lincoln was at the time reputed to be the best chiropractic school in the United States. My skepticism about chiropractic theory notwithstanding, I must say that our curriculum and instructors were first rate. We were even schooled in nutrition, a subject that would not be taught regularly in most medical schools until decades later. Most of the first two years were heavily classroom oriented, focusing on the same hard sciences (anatomy, chemistry) required of medical school students, as well as Lincoln chiropractic theory and office procedures, such as physical examination and treatment techniques—the main one being manipulation. During the second phase of our studies, we mixed classroom work with participation in the mandatory two-year clinical program. There we saw real patients, just like medical school interns.

The Anatomy of Lincolnian Chiropractic

Before I summarize what I learned at Lincoln about chiropractic diagnosis and treatment, let me identify and describe for your benefit the main anatomical focus of chiropractic, the spinal column, and a few other anatomical features.

The spine is made up of several sections of bony structures called vertebrae. These vertebrae are aligned vertically and separated from each other by circular spongy pads of tissue called discs. These discs serve as shock absorbers to prevent the vertebrae from coming into contact with the spinal cord, which could cause paralysis or death.

The sections of the spine, from top to bottom, are known as the atlas and axis, the rest of the cervical spine, the thoracic spine, and the lumbar spine. The lumbar spine rests on an arrowhead-shaped bone called the sacrum, which is composed of a number of separate sections fused together. The sacrum is important because attached to it on each side is an illium, the half-moon shaped bone commonly known as the hipbone. The coccyx, or tailbone, is attached to the bottom of the sacrum.

The human skull rests on the top two vertebrae of the cervical (neck) portion of the spine, called the atlas and the axis. The atlas, a ring-shaped bone, rests upon the axis, a post-like structure. The ring of the atlas revolves around the post of the axis, thereby allowing the head to rotate from side to side, as well as up and down.

The remaining vertebrae in the cervical as well as in the thoracic (upper back) and lumbar (lower back) sections of the spine resemble each other more than they do the atlas or axis. These vertebrae vary in size depending on their location in the spine, or spinal column. Each vertebra features a bony, knob-like projection on the back called the spinous process, and from both the left and right sides of each vertebra protrudes another bony, knob-like projection called the transverse process. On a person with minimal body fat on the backside, you can see the outline of and feel the spinous processes underneath the skin. The spinous processes and transverse processes of the vertebrae are attached to spinal muscles, which serve to keep the vertebrae vertically aligned.

The spinal cord begins at the base of the brain and runs downward. It then passes through the center of the spinal canal, which runs through the center of each of the vertebrae in the spinal column. The spinal cord ends at the sacrum. From both the left and right side of each vertebra, a nerve branches out from the spinal cord. Each of these spinal cord nerves continues on to a specific organ, muscle, or system in the body, providing nerve energy to those areas. Nerves from each side of the sacrum also branch out to the lower part of the body.

The Lincoln Fork in the Road

Whether you walk into a medical clinic or a chiropractor's office with back pain, your goal is the same: get rid of it. The difference between the Lincoln Chiropractic interns and medical interns was what they believed caused the back pain, and how to get rid of it. My Lincoln Clinic patients said that their medical doctors had told them that their back pain was caused by a slipped disk, rheumatism, or arthritis. Medically, this left them with two treatment options: pain killers or surgery.

At Lincoln, we were taught that when a "stress" either from within the body or from outside the body causes a given vertebra to shift, or subluxate, from its normal position, the vertebra will pinch the spinal cord nerve, inhibiting the flow of nerve energy to a particular organ, muscle, or system in the body. The resulting pain, numbness, or malfunction is known as the "pinched nerve effect." To this day, this explanation is probably still accepted by a majority of chiropractors. Thus, we agreed with the medical doctors insofar as the possibility that a pinched nerve could cause back or neck pain. The difference was that, according to chiropractic theory, the nerve being pinched, as well as what was pinching it, could be identified and the problem could be resolved without drugs or surgery.

So what could cause an internal stress? Since the only thing attached to the vertebra is muscle, then slippage of the vertebra from an internal stress would have to be caused by muscle. My instructors at Lincoln offered no explanation as to how or why this could happen, and it remained a mystery to me for several years. Identifying external forces that could cause slippage was easier: falls, straining, or trauma were the usual suspects.

In the end, though, the issue of whether internal or external forces caused the slippage didn't really matter to us, as our main concern in the Lincoln clinic was how to locate and fix it.

The Lincoln Clinic

The Lincoln Chiropractic College in Indianapolis, was located in a nice area of town in a single large building. Lincoln's clinical program was located in an area on the first floor, and operated Monday through Friday. All interns in the Clinical program worked a two-hour shift on each of those days, and the rest of our time was spent attending classes.

Aside from the fact that treatment to all patients was free of charge, it was not clear how patients ended up at the Lincoln Clinic.

One thing their histories had in common, though, was unsuccessful treatment of neck or back pain by medical doctors.

Our individual patients were initially screened by the Clinic Director, who assigned them to the interns. While according to theory we could apply chiropractic treatment principles to anything from asthma to vision problems, the patients we saw usually complained of neck or back pain.

Once we met with our new patients in one of the treatment rooms, we would check their vital signs and take their histories. We then performed a physical exam, including a visual exam and palpation of the spine, which meant that we examined the spine with our hands. The main purpose of palpation was to locate subluxation in the spine by feel. We palpated the cervical and thoracic spines in a sitting position and palpated the lumbar spine with the patient lying face down on a specially designed table called an adjustment table. The examination could also include X-rays, which would help identify a subluxated vertebra. We ordered X-rays only about 25% to 35% of the time, as we were concerned about patients getting too much exposure to radiation.

After taking into consideration the history, physical exam, X-rays, and all other relevant factors, we made a decision within the guidelines we were given in class how to proceed with treatment. For example, we had been taught that when a patient experiences pain in the neck, we should suspect subluxation in the cervical spine. For pain in the low back or leg, we had been taught to suspect subluxation of the lumbar/sacrum or sacrum/iliac joint. When the patient complained of malfunction in an organ or other area of the body, we were told to suspect subluxation of the vertebra(e) closest to the nerve(s) supplying energy to that organ or area of the body.

Once we located the subluxation, the mandatory chiropractic treatment was manipulation, also more commonly known to our patients as an "adjustment." Manipulation was the use of our hands at the site of the subluxation in a thrusting motion in an attempt to literally push the subluxated vertebra or sacrum back into its normal position. First we did a general manipulation, to loosen or stretch muscles in preparation for the second, more vertebra-specific manipulation. As we manipulated, we were to listen for cracking or popping noises, which usually indicated that the subluxated vertebra or sacrum had returned to its normal position. Sometimes we would even be able to feel the vertebra or sacrum move back into place.

If, after manipulation, the pain lessened or disappeared, the manipulation was said to have "held." We could then assume that we had restored the subluxated vertebra or sacrum to its normal position, thereby eliminating the pinching of the affected nerve and allowing nerve energy to flow once again to the affected organ, muscle, or body system.

If, after the manipulation, however, the pain did not disappear or subside, or worsened, our response would be that the manipulation did not hold, meaning that the subluxated vertebra had shifted only partially or not at all back into its normal position. If asked why the manipulation did not hold, our response was to be that we didn't know, or that the patient had unwittingly done something to prevent it from holding. In this event, the patient willing, we would usually attempt multiple additional manipulations over days, weeks, or months, perhaps taking additional X-rays to track our progress.

If additional manipulations didn't resolve the patient's problems, orthodox chiropractic had, at that time, nothing further to offer in the way of treatment. The so-called "modalities," such as ultrasound or "cold quartz" treatments were offered to supplement or facilitate manipulation, but not as alternatives to manipulation. Thus, a patient who failed to get relief from medical practitioners and chiropractors had three basic alternatives: put up with the pain (often accompanied by loss of range of movement and functionality), take pain medication, or consult with an orthopedic surgeon.

At this point, you may be wondering if I fared any better in the Lincoln clinic than in my early Buffalo practice. The answer is, unfortunately, no, I didn't get results there, either. You might say that what I did get was a severe case of clinical disappointment.

Most of the patients assigned to me in the Lincoln clinic had low back or sacroiliac problems, for which, modalities aside, I had only manipulation to offer. Unfortunately, manipulation provided token, temporary, or no relief. As for those patients whose lumbar or sacral manipulations held the first time, their pain often returned shortly thereafter—but they did not. Worse yet, for those patients I saw with cervical pain, manipulation seldom held.

I experienced a growing fear that, despite all I had been taught, physical reality did not live up to Lincoln, or any other, chiropractic theory. I began to question whether pain and sickness really were the result of a nerve pinched by a subluxated vertebra, or something else. The last straw of doubt came to me in the form of positive results I achieved with a Lincoln Clinic patient by using no chiropractic at all.

One day, a male asthmatic patient was assigned to me. Emboldened by a lack of results with manipulation, I was inspired to deviate from the mandatory manipulation and approach his problem with a different technique: nutrition. Partly from my knowledge on nutrition and partly from intuition, I simply told him to refrain from eating all dairy, flour, and sugar products. I administered no manipulation, no ultrasound.

Within two weeks, he was responding very well. Not only had his breathing improved, but the severity of his other symptoms not associated with asthma had decreased. He was having fewer and less severe headaches, as well as less fatigue. I instructed him to stay on this diet. A few days later, however, I happened to run into him—in a bakery—with his hand literally in the cookie jar. He apologized to me, saying that he couldn't help it, that he constantly craved sugar. Understandably, he didn't show up for his next appointment.

Though I lost my asthmatic patient to an addiction I did not then understand, the experience was nonetheless revelatory. Having witnessed the unreliability of manipulation on so many external problems, I concluded that the theory underlying chiropractic was invalid for internal problems, too. I felt that my studies now qualified me to pass judgment on the validity of chiropractic theory and practice, and I was no longer willing to distract myself from doubt by drawing analogies to conventional medical practice as "different strokes for different folks." However, for the time being I returned my focus to doing whatever was necessary to graduate, and pushed to the back of my mind the scary thought of how I would deal with lack of results once I entered practice.

CHAPTER 3
Buffaloed In Buffalo

I started my practice in Buffalo in 1950 in a rented second-story office, where I saw patients in the evenings after working at Sylvania Electronics all day. As had been the case at the Lincoln Clinic, most of my patients had already been to a medical doctor for lumbar or sacroiliac pain, and were told they had rheumatism, a slipped disc or arthritis. Chiropractic was their last hope for drugless, non-surgical resolution.

During my first year or two in practice, I attempted to increase my success rate with manipulation by modifying the lumbar-sacral and sacroiliac manipulation I learned at Lincoln, and a few patients began to get well. Overall, though, chiropractic was not working as I'd been led to believe, despite my rigorous adherence to applying what I was taught. I felt that I was alone in a desperate situation. I was rapidly losing faith in the basic tenets of my profession in a world where few people had even heard of chiropractic. I didn't receive support from my friends or family. I couldn't brainstorm with the few other chiropractors in Buffalo because none of them had been trained in Lincoln's methods. I could buy some time with my day job, but I knew that eventually I would either have to make chiropractic work for me, or try to climb the corporate ladder at Sylvania.

As I had experienced it, manipulation was a technique in search of a supporting theory. My knowledge of physiology and anatomy tempted me to buy into the pinched nerve effect, at least for musculoskeletal problems, but not for asthmatics, and probably not for other internal problems. Though I had actually verified the existence of and realigned subluxated lumbar and sacral joints, these results were often short-lived. Manipulation in the cervical spines held even less frequently. If at all possible, I needed to find out why manipulation, the main weapon in the arsenal of chiropractic treatment, wasn't working.

The answer, I told myself, might be found by returning to the point at which chiropractic theory began and delving deeper into the details of what I was taught were the causes of subluxation—internal or external "stress." How did muscles, the only anatomically logical or possible source of internal stress, cause a vertebra to subluxate? The instructors at Lincoln didn't know. Also, were trauma, straining, and falls really the so-called external stresses that caused subluxation? I told myself that if I could answer these questions, I could answer other important questions: Was manipulation really the solution for subluxation? In other words, if what I'd been taught at Lincoln about the cause of subluxation was not fully understood, or was just plain wrong, where did that leave manipulation as the basis for an entire philosophy of treatment? I decided to do to the musculoskeletal system what I had done to my toys and to radar equipment in the military: take it apart, and see how it worked. This, I felt, was the best way to figure out how to fix it.

To begin with, I reasoned that if palpation helped me locate a subluxated vertebra it might give me clues to what caused the vertebra to subluxate in the first place, as well as what sets this process in motion, whether from within or without the body. Atherosclerosis, for example, is a process. It doesn't appear or become life-threatening overnight. It takes a while. Medicine found the cause by identifying and understanding the process of its development and working backwards from there to find what sets that process in motion; for example, diet.

Besides failing to give us information about the cause or mechanics of subluxation, the instructors at Lincoln didn't tell us how long it took for a vertebra to subluxate. Was it a discrete event—one moment you're fine, the next you've been subluxated? Or was it progressive, like atherosclerosis, taking possibly weeks, months, or years to develop? Also, was there pain during the entire slippage process—however long it took—or only after a certain degree of slippage? As students, we were never told if the degree of subluxation we palpated or saw on X-rays was at its theoretical maximum, or still an ongoing process. If a patient's subluxation were left untreated, would X-rays a year later reveal the same degree of displacement, or an even greater one? With these questions as my analytical wallpaper, I began my quest.

At Lincoln, we never were taught to use palpation anywhere but on the spine. After all, subluxation had meaning only for the spine, and the only purpose of palpation was to locate the subluxation through the sense of touch. It was clear to me that I would, in my use of palpation, have to think outside the spine, focusing no longer on the subluxated vertebra, but on the condition of the muscles and skin surrounding the vertebra.

So it was that around the end of my second year of practice in Buffalo, I began palpating outside of the spine for clues. I palpated the muscles adjacent to areas of the lumbar spine and sacrum in which there were complaints of pain—something we never did at Lincoln. When I did so, I noticed that these areas felt warmer to the touch than areas where there had been no complaints of pain.

Also, the surface of the muscle tissue adjacent to these same complaint areas often felt different—lumpy, knotty, or rippled— whereas other, non-complaint areas felt smoother to the touch. Soon I began to develop increased sensitivity in my fingertips, which allowed me to feel more precisely these differences in the muscle tissue. This increased sensitivity was greatly amplified by my use of a particular lubricant. I found that by rubbing it on a given area before palpating, I was able to feel with tremendously greater precision the differences in tissue "topography." Remarkably this substance, which I started using in the 1950's, has been continuously manufactured since that time, if not earlier, and I still use it.

Paralleling my developing tactile sensitivity was the training of my eyes to spot differences in the contour of the skin created by the underlying muscle tissue in the complaint areas, as compared to non-complaint areas. Some areas were unnaturally rounder or flatter than others.

At that point I didn't know the cause or significance of these relative variations in temperature and topography of the tissues between complaint and non-complaint areas. Were they clues to the nature of the internal stress said to cause subluxation? I couldn't say then, but I knew these variations weren't normal. The fact that they consistently corresponded with the boundaries between complaint and non-complaint areas appeared to be more than mere coincidence. I felt that I was onto something, but exactly what or how big I would not know for a while. I also didn't know at the time that, by developing these comparative palpation and visual examination techniques, I had abandoned the path of ignorance and entered the on-ramp to positive epiphanies.

In Kneed of an Epiphany

By 1952 I had been in practice for almost two years, and my sense of urgency to make chiropractic work for me was heightened by the birth of my son. Though initially encouraged by the comparative palpation and visual examination techniques I had developed, I began to grow impatient. My intuition told me that the variations in muscle tissue revealed by these techniques were important clues to the cause or process of subluxation. But what was missing? What more did I need to make use of these clues in practice? I didn't know it, but I was on the verge of experiencing my first epiphany, and it would have nothing to do with the spinal column.

At that time, I couldn't afford X-ray equipment, so I had farmed out that task to a retired chiropractor from the Palmer school by the name of Dr. Walton. He and a fellow Lincoln graduate,

Dr. Harold Dahlstrom, were the only peers I had encountered
in Buffalo. I came to know Walton better over time, and later
developed a loose friendship with Dahlstrom, who, along with
Walton, would unwittingly send me down the path of epiphanies.

One day Walton offered to give me a piece of equipment from
his former practice. This "equipment," a dark-colored wooden chair
with a wide, deep, flat seat and an armrest on each side, was foreign
to my experience. The seat was unusually high off the floor, so unless
you were extremely tall, your legs didn't touch the floor when seated.
He explained to me that he had used it for examining knees, but he
did not explain how he examined them, what he looked for, or what
he did when he found it. His failure to offer any more information
was not unusual, since he did not discuss much about his former
practice, and I didn't ask. At any rate, this exam chair immediately
aroused my curiosity. Figuring I had nothing to lose, and that I
might need it some day, I accepted the chair.

Up to this point, the majority of my patients complained
of lumbar or sacroiliac pain. Next most frequent were cervical
problems. The few remaining patients I saw had a mix of knee, hip,
shoulder, ankle, elbow, and foot problems. I also had been exploring
these areas with my comparative palpation and visual exams.

One day, not long after I took possession of my gift exam chair,
a patient with a knee problem came to me, and I decided to examine
the patient in my new chair. As I had done with my previous
knee patients, I palpated the knee joint and all the muscles in the
surrounding area and, as usual, I detected differences in temperature
in different areas in and around the joint as well as differences in
how the muscle tissue felt in one area compared to others. I noted
that the problem knee joint looked somewhat deformed.

I continued examining the patient in the chair with his leg
extended toward me, while I straddled his leg with my legs, facing
him. Of all the areas of the body outside the spine, I had been
studying in particular and had become most familiar with the knee.
From what I saw of this patient, I felt there was subluxation in the
knee joint, and wondered if it could be manipulated back into place.

In an attempt to prepare the knee for manipulation, I began to stretch and, in some sense of the word, massage the muscles around the joint. Then, somewhat intuitively and somewhat experimentally, I grasped the knee joint with both hands and attempted to move it in a combined rotating and pushing fashion, like a crank. All at once, the patient and I both heard a muffled popping sound. I held my breath. After a few seconds of silence, I began re-examining the knee. The patient said the pain was gone. My examination revealed that the joint looked normal again, and I felt a great reduction of the inflammation and swelling of the muscles and the joint in general. These changes and the patient's feedback confirmed to me what I had already suspected: I had performed a successful manipulation of his subluxated knee joint, returning it to normal.

If my patient was impressed, he didn't show it. No doubt he expected his good result, as if that's what was supposed to happen when you go to a chiropractor. I, however, was stunned. Though at the time I didn't even know the word "epiphany" existed, I later realized that I had experienced a major one.

This was a momentous occasion for me and my practice for two reasons. First, contrary to all chiropractic schools of thought, it was clear that at least one subluxated joint outside the spinal column could be manipulated back into its normal position. Whether or not it would work with other joints remained to be seen, since I had been focusing on the knee in particular.

Secondly, while this phenomenon didn't explain why manipulation didn't always work, or what caused the subluxation, the post-manipulation disappearance of swelling, inflammation, and disparities in the affected knee and leg made it clear that these symptoms were involved in whatever process that was responsible for subluxation in the first place.

As I'm sure you can understand, this epiphany profoundly affected me in another way. I lost another quantum of my already fading faith in chiropractic. According to Lincoln, manipulation of any joint outside the spine was not even to be considered, let alone possible! According to Lincoln, I should not have been able to do what I did, or get the results I did, without manipulating the spine.

However, not only did I do it, but I consistently and easily would reproduce that result on many, many more knee patients, among others, during the next 43 years of my practice.

If what I learned at Lincoln about how chiropractic could fix knee problems was wrong, where else was my chiropractic education flawed? I suppose that one who was not in the desperate situation I was in could have looked at what happened in a more positive, philosophical way: that it was but another refinement on theory, or a tweak on technique, another mile marker in the evolution of chiropractic, as was the creation of Lincoln as a school that taught manipulation of the whole spine. However, I couldn't afford the luxury of philosophizing. I felt I was under the gun to investigate which aspects of chiropractic theory and treatment were valid and which were not, which were salvageable and which were not, in order to make a critical decision about my career that would affect my ability to support my family.

Eventually, the euphoria I experienced with my first successful manipulation of the knee again gave way to impatience. What had been a new height for me developed into a years-long plateau akin to limbo. For the next eight or so years in Buffalo, I languished as I stared at the wall separating me from the missing links of knowledge I was certain lay on the other side—the information necessary to make a living out of chiropractic. Eventually, as with many who grow stale professionally, I decided it was time to seek out inspiration from a change of scenery, and began preparing to relocate my practice to the beautiful bluegrass and hills of Kentucky. . .or so I thought.

It was around this time that I received a call from Dr. Harold Dahlstrom. I had shortly before suggested to him that he practice in Indiana. Ironically, he now told me about a chiropractor named Dr. Paul Nolting in Indiana who had two practices for sale, one in Indianapolis, and one in a small city about 30 miles southeast of Indianapolis, Shelbyville. Since my memories of living in Indy while attending Lincoln were positive and I held licenses to practice not only in Kentucky, but in Vermont and Indiana, I decided to take a scouting trip to Shelbyville.

One important factor in deciding to buy any practice was whether or not it could support my family. When I arrived there in early 1959, I was comforted to find that Shelbyville, the county seat of this primarily farming region of Hoosier Land, had two banks, a General Electric plant, a plastic bag factory, a new library, a new high school, and was to be situated alongside a new stretch of highway called Interstate 74, which would connect Shelbyville and Indianapolis. The practice came with a large base of 200 existing patients, which was the most important factor in my decision. This told me that the people of Shelbyville were not alien to chiropractic care and would be receptive to my presence in the community. However, it was an additional plus that Dr. Nolting was also a Lincoln graduate, as the patients would be assured that the treatment techniques they were accustomed to would continue with the new doctor. Thus fortified by these positive signs, I purchased the Shelbyville practice from Dr. Nolting, who later became my friend.

My family—especially my mother—was not exactly happy about the move. Instead of "Nino, where did you come from?" she now asked, "Nino, where are you going?" Even more puzzling to her than what it was that I did for a living was the fact that I was moving 500 miles from Buffalo to do it. I, at least, absolutely knew where I was going and why. What no one could know at the time was what additional epiphanies were awaiting me in Shelbyville.

CHAPTER 4
Saving Dr. Ramsey

I had hoped that opening my Shelbyville practice at 17 East Broadway in September 1959 would invigorate and inspire me as I renewed my effort to provide a living for my family by getting results in my office.

Along with my new office address, there was a change of my family name. Though certainly proud of my Sicilian heritage and family name Ippolito, I had been worried about how that name might sound to a patient base in rural Indiana, which, rightly or wrongly, I assumed to be less ethnically diversified than Buffalo. I knew that for many, Ippolito would not be easy to spell or pronounce, and I wondered about what effect any possible negative perceptions about my ethnicity might have on my efforts to maintain and build the practice I had just purchased.

My wife, who was born in Chicago but grew up in Indiana, was certain that a name she picked out would be more ethnically acceptable to this small community in the heartland of America. Thus, much to the further dismay of my mother, a court in Erie County, New York changed our family name. When I opened my new office in Shelbyville I introduced myself as Dr. John A. Ramsey to the new patients who were already waiting for me at the door.

The practice I purchased from Dr. Paul Nolting consisted of a few pieces of office furniture and equipment, including an adjustment table, and his patient files. The rented office containing this practice, flanked by a restaurant and a bar, consisted of a storefront-window waiting room facing the main street, a center exam/treatment room, a small private office, and a bathroom.

For whatever reason, Paul and I never discussed whether or not he and I had common frustrations in getting results. At any rate, during the first few months, I advanced no further in getting results than I had in Buffalo—same plateau, different zip code. In a final act of desperation, I even purchased a standard modality instrument: an ultrasound machine. I was not surprised to find that it did nothing to improve my situation.

Less than a year old, my fresh start already felt stale. I was simultaneously at the end of my rope and a fork in the road. To the left lay some other way to make a living and support my family. To the right, one last all-out, no-holds-barred effort to find the missing links to consistently successful treatment of joint and back pain— with manipulation if possible, or without if necessary. Lincoln had schooled me in the art of manipulation, but it was unreliable. At any rate, it was a form of treatment, not diagnosis.

I wasn't ready to take the left fork. I was determined to make chiropractic—or something like it—work for me, and that was that. As I then sized up the situation, I needed to "retro-diagnose" subluxation—trace it back to its beginning and identify the essential elements of the process—thereby, I hoped, understanding how manipulation fit into the overall picture. Anybody could be trained to locate and perform manipulation on a subluxated vertebra. The real question was, why didn't it always work? This question logically gave way to another, even more basic one: Was manipulation really the right tool in the first place?

As I assessed the best way to retro-diagnose, I recalled my first successful manipulation of the knee. The experience proved to me the value of my comparative visual and palpation exam techniques, so it seemed logical to start with them in developing my retro-diagnostic procedures. The problem was figuring out how to use them. The inspiration for the answer came in the form of an article by a chiropractor discussing "muscle testing." I can't recall much about the article now, but I recall that it made me think: did the relative strength or weakness of a muscle or muscle group in a joint play a role in the process of subluxation?

I came away from my first knee manipulation with the thought that the clumsy, unprincipled massage I had performed on the muscles in the knee joint had contributed to the success of the manipulation. After all, we had been taught to stretch the spinal muscles in preparation for manipulation, so, why not the muscles involved in the joints, too? I concluded that the integrity of the knee joint could not be viewed in isolation. The relative health of the muscles involved in the normal functioning of that joint must likewise influence the subluxation of that joint.

Recognizing that the cardinal test for the relative health of a muscle is how well it contracts and relaxes, I decided to experiment with massage of the muscles involved in a given joint to see if there were differences between their pre- and post-massage performance. At the same time it occurred to me that, helpful as my comparative visual and palpation techniques had been so far, I would have to modify them for retro-diagnosis. In order for my practice to thrive, I would have to think outside the box just as I had during an emergency situation I had experienced during World War II.

While stationed in Okinawa, I was the sergeant in charge of the crew responsible for operating and maintaining the Ground Control Approach or "GCA." This radar equipment transmitted a signal to the incoming planes that helped our pilots land safely. On one occasion, I was awakened in the middle of the night and told that an approaching squadron of U.S. fighter planes was running low on fuel and needed to land at our base. When I gathered my crew and attempted to activate the GCA, we couldn't get it to transmit. We tried everything in the procedure manual to no avail. The situation was growing critical. If we didn't fix the problem soon, the pilots would have to ditch in the ocean. As I frantically tried to figure out what was wrong, I suddenly remembered that it had rained the night before. Despite the fact that no such scenario was mentioned in the

GCA equipment troubleshooting manual, I decided to check to see if the rainwater could somehow be responsible. I took my men outside the trailer housing us and our electronics and began to inspect the GCA equipment. We found that the Wave Guide, a rectangular metal box-like device that transmitted radio waves to the transmitting antenna, was full of rainwater. Theoretically, this water could short-circuit the electronics. We emptied the Wave Guide, dried it, and again attempted to activate the GCA. This time it worked like a charm, and the planes were able to land safely.

Inspired by the same kind of thought process that got us out of that jam, I expanded my increasingly efficient comparative visual and palpation exams outward from the portions of the muscles nearest the joint, and eventually to entire regions of the body, beginning with the joints of the upper and lower extremities—the arms from the tips of the fingers to the shoulder, and the legs from the buttocks to the ends of the toes and the heels.

As my exams branched out to the extremities, I also began to massage these areas as well, along the way transforming my crude massage strokes into efficient, highly effective techniques for loosening taut muscles. At the same time, I devised my own muscle testing techniques, which eventually gave me clues not only to the nature of the subluxation process, but to the true cause of joint pain.

Over the next year or so, I became proficient in developing joint-specific manipulation techniques and consistently performing successful manipulations in the shoulder, elbow, wrist, hand, finger, knee, ankle, foot, and toe. Without exception, a successful manipulation in the affected joint would result in the immediate cessation of pain, a reduction in swelling and inflammation, and the resumption of normal functioning of the joint. What I found during this period was that the knee and the other non-spinal subluxated joints can, when properly prepared, be manipulated back into place.

Despite these successes I still had a long way to go, retro-diagnostically speaking. While I was safe for the moment concluding that the subluxation process for all these joints was probably the same, I still didn't know the how, why, or when of the process. Yes, I knew that the muscles involved in a given painful joint were taut, swollen, and inflamed. And, yes, I knew that my massage of these muscles helped prepare the joint for a successful manipulation. I just didn't understand exactly what in the subluxation process was causing these symptoms and the very need for manipulation—if manipulation were needed at all. For diagnosing back and neck pain, Lincoln taught me to suspect subluxation of one or more vertebrae in the spine and manipulate accordingly. Although the realization was perhaps long overdue, I had another epiphany during this period that, in my mind, invalidated this tenet of chiropractic.

One day, I was treating a patient for low back pain. In order to steady myself for an attempt at manipulation, I rested one of my palms between his shoulder blades, while I used my other hand to perform the manipulation on his low back. As I shifted my position, I unconsciously applied additional weight to the palm in between his shoulder blades. Just then both he and I heard and felt one of his vertebrae slipping back into position. I asked him if he had ever felt any pain in between his shoulder blades before, after or during this event, and he said that he had not.

I then remembered that this was not the first time I had witnessed this phenomenon or heard about it from a patient. Many patients had recalled such a muffled "pop" and painless sensation of vertebral movement during stretching or other movements. Then there were the patients who had constant pain when not moving, or when taking a breath, or where there were no displaced vertebrae. I then flashed back to the many times I had noticed subluxated vertebrae in X-rays, yet received no complaint of pain from the patient in the area of the subluxation.

The critical epiphany here was that, contrary to what I was taught at Lincoln, subluxated vertebrae are not the source, cause, or location of the pain—it was the spinal muscles that were painful!

In the wake of this realization I would find that, with the muscles of the joints as well as in the spine, uneven tension in the muscles in one side would, over time, begin to pull the vertebra or bone into subluxation. In my experience, subluxation in the cervical and lumbar spines took the form of rotation to either side, or slippage both posteriorly (backwards) and inferiorly (downwards) or, in some cases, both rotationally and posteriorly. Regardless, as it began to subluxate, the vertebra would shift in the direction from which came the greater pull. With the spine, depending on how long the disparity in muscle tension had existed, it might take only minimal massage of the muscles attached to this vertebra to relax the muscles on the tighter side to allow the vertebra to slip back into its normal position, either during an attempt at manipulation, or spontaneously, as the result of sudden movement. It was now clear to me why some manipulations held and others didn't. In some cases, where the uneven pull was minimal and of short duration, the vertebra was a manipulation waiting to happen, even without preparation of the muscles by stretching. Again, I remembered hearing patients describe spontaneous manipulation resulting simply from their turning one way or the other. It was just as clear to me now that, in the case where the uneven pulling had been present for some time and the degree and extent of tautness was severe, manipulation would either not happen, or not hold. Successful conscious manipulations were in essence inadvertent, more the result of good timing than good technique. That being the case, manipulation of the spine was unnecessary, and I discarded it, except in rare circumstances.

At this point, you may be asking, "Why was manipulation necessary for joints in the extremities, but unnecessary for subluxation in the spine?" The answer, as I see it, lies in the difference in the musculature and the nature of the joints, compared to that of the spine. The vertebrae, on one hand, are supported and held in place by a tremendously powerful and comparatively massive set of muscles. The muscles involved in the joints of the extremities, however—even in the knee—are not nearly as massive, strong, or stabilizing, so the joints in the extremities are not as stable. Also, I believe that, since the muscle mass in the spinal area is so much greater, it takes correspondingly more time, even with massage, for the spinal muscles to relax to the degree necessary to allow the vertebra to slip back into place—with manipulation or without.

I couldn't help shaking my head as I contemplated the irony in this epiphany: Lincoln taught me to manipulate only the spine, and not the joints of the extremities. Yet, contrary to what I was taught, manipulation was, in my experience, not only unreliable and unnecessary for spinal subluxation, but mandatory for painful joints—for which it was never intended!

So, how had my collective epiphanies shaped my opinion about the validity of chiropractic theory and practice? As concerned my practice, the coffin of chiropractic theory and practice had been pretty much been nailed shut. True, Lincoln had given me manipulation, but I used it only for non-spinal subluxation. And yes…Lincoln had also given me palpation, a skill which I had developed and found very useful—and would eventually find indispensable.

On balance, though, it was clear to me that, in the short term, back pain, joint pain, and disease were NOT caused by a subluxated vertebra. To the contrary, though diagnostically helpful, a subluxated vertebra is relatively insignificant unless or until it threatens the spinal cord or the nerves that branch out from the cord.

I felt like a Phoenix rising from my initial failures to achieve success with chiropractic and reeducating myself out of desperation. Yet my re-education was far from over, and my professional salvation far from complete. With all the progress I had made down the right fork in the road, I still needed answers to some crucial questions, including: What causes the pronounced, uneven muscle tension involved in subluxation in the spine and extremities? During the next few decades, I would be amazed at the answers I found through two final major epiphanies.

CHAPTER 5
A Long Walk On A Short Leg

Have you ever looked either at yourself or another person and noticed that one body part or area in some way looked different than its counterpart? For example, one arm or one hand looking bigger than the other? Or one calf being thicker or having a different shape than the other? If so, you were observing what is called "asymmetry," or a lack of symmetry. By asymmetry, I mean that one object of a pair is different than its counterpart in terms of size, position, shape, or in other ways I'll describe shortly.

If you did notice a lack of symmetry on yourself or someone else, what did you think about it? Did you wonder about what, if anything, it meant, or why or how it came to be, or whether it resulted from birth, well-concealed surgery, perhaps an injury? One last question: Did you ever wonder if it could be made symmetrical?

I briefly mentioned in Chapter 4 that, in developing my comparative visual and palpation exam techniques, I found and wondered about the significance of certain dissimilarities or asymmetries in my patients. It was during this period that not only was I developing and refining my palpation, massage, and joint manipulation techniques, but I was also improving my ability to spot asymmetries crucial to identifying the areas to muscle test and massage prior to manipulation.

I based my comparative visual exams for asymmetry on the assumption that the size, position, shape, and relative location of anatomical structures or features on the left side of a patient's body should mirror those on the right. If they didn't, I reasoned, the abnormal side was a clue to the cause of the patient's troubles. Eventually, once I identified the abnormal side, the rest was a matter of massage and manipulation.

I didn't just compare areas of the body to see if they looked the same, I also searched for what I'll call "tactile" symmetry. Even if both features of a pair of anatomical structures or features looked symmetrical, I palpated them to see if they felt the same. Were both sides smooth to the touch, or one soft and the other knotty or taut? Were both sides roughly the same temperature (cool to the touch is normal), or was one warmer to the touch?

Once I determined that one structure or area looked and/or felt abnormal, I stepped back and viewed the entire region of the body to see if I could relate the proximity of the abnormal side to the area of the painful joint or site.

As I became more proficient in successfully diagnosing and manipulating subluxation in the joints of the extremities, a key factor in my success was my growing ability to identify asymmetry along the entire upper and lower extremities, both in the visual and tactile senses. I was surprised to see an incredible amount of asymmetry not only in my patients, but also in people on the street. It's amazing what you can see when you know what to look for, and equally amazing how widespread these asymmetries seemed to be.

I discerned several types of asymmetry from which I would soon be able to put the pieces of the subluxation puzzle together. First, there were variations in size. For example, even taking into account such obvious factors as "dominant hand" or weight training, one of the calves or thighs would have a greater diameter, or one hand or arm would be larger. More subtle were variations in the diameter of the ankle or size of the heel. Or, when I would have a patient sit in a chair, one knee would be closer to the edge of the seat.

Next were variations in contour or fullness. One side of a patient's face would have a swollen appearance as compared to the other; a patient's rib cage, clavicle, or scapula would protrude or "stick out" more on one side than the other. A woman's right breast might be lower or higher than the left, or fuller, or flatter, or pointing more to one side than straight ahead. One of the calves or buttocks would have a flat spot, as opposed to the other, which would be perfectly rounded, or one buttock might have a dimple.

Next was a category of asymmetry focusing on length, height, or position. For example, a patient's left shoulder might be thrusting forward while the right shoulder was thrusting back. The vertical measurement of the neck between the head and the shoulder might be longer on one side than the other, or the length of the abdomen between the bottom of the rib cage and the hip might be longer on one side. A patient's head might be rotated clockwise or counter-clockwise, or might be ever so slightly tilted to the left or right side. Looking at the patient straight in the face, you could see that one ear is closer to the front of his head than the other. The patient's chest could be sunken, the shoulders might be rounded, or it could even appear that the patient's head was being drawn into his chest, much like a turtle's head is retracted into its shell. One knee cap could be pointing slightly to one side instead of straight ahead; one or more of the patient's toes on one foot may be abnormally curled to the side; the arches of the feet may be different. And all of these irregularities existed almost entirely unbeknownst to the patients.

Because my comparative exam is based upon the principle that everything on both sides of the patient's body should both look and feel the same, I found it useful to refer to differences in relative temperature or topography as asymmetry as well. Thus, there are "tactile" asymmetries: for example, one side or area of one thigh muscle might be abnormally warm to the touch, or much tighter than the opposing side; it might be swollen. Then there is what I'll call "functional" asymmetry: for example, one leg or one arm would be stronger than the other, even accounting for the "dominant limb" factor. Or a patient would display marked differences in the way that he or she moved one leg in comparison to the other while walking. Finally, there was asymmetry in sensitivity: one area might be painful to the touch, but not painful in use; one of a woman's breasts may be far more tender than the other; one ankle or one arm or thigh might not hurt in use, but might be tender to the touch; one side of the jaw or cheek may evidence no pain until the patient chews or yawns; there may also be tension in the teeth in one or more quadrants compared to the others, or sensitivity in the mouth or gums, even where dental disease has been ruled out.

During my 45 years of practice, I repeatedly observed in my patients every example of asymmetry I have listed here and more. In my experience, each of them has been and continues to be diagnostically significant to me to one degree or another regarding pain, subluxation, loss of range of motion, or disease that the patient is either already experiencing, or will likely experience in the future, given certain assumptions, which I will detail later.

During the more than five years I spent at the Broadway office, I further developed and polished some very effective retro-diagnostic tools, such as comparative visual and palpation exams to identify various types of asymmetry, as well as muscle testing, massage, and joint-specific manipulation. As I became more proficient in the use of these tools, I developed yet another. It was a key diagnostic tool that built upon the others and helped accelerate me down the right fork in high gear: the ability to spot recurrent patterns.

One of the first patterns I discovered related to pain in the sacroiliac joint. As you'll remember, the sacrum is the arrowhead-shaped bone consisting, for my purposes, of two sections, "S-1" and "S-2." The sacrum, upon which rests the fifth, or lowest, lumbar vertebra, "L-5," is attached on each side to the half-moon-shaped bone called the ilium, more commonly known as the hip bone. Inserted into each ilium bone is a femur, the long bone of the upper leg. The area where the sacrum and the ilium are joined, like several others in the body, is very unstable, and is one of the most common sites of lower back pain. "Why?" I asked myself. As I looked more closely at the problem, I asked myself another question: Why, far more often than not, did the pain occur only on one side—the right? Patterned asymmetry in the legs and knee joints would later provide me with clues.

There were other recurring examples of patterned asymmetry, as well. For example, complaints of neck or shoulder pain would always be accompanied by a variety of asymmetries in the neck, scapula (shoulder blade), clavicle (collarbone), and other areas, and, again, would usually be limited to one side of the body. Also, knee problems would evidence asymmetry in the muscles surrounding the problem knee—but often on that knee only. Foot pain, whether underneath the arch, on top of the foot, in the heel, or in the toes, also would usually be limited to one side and accompanied by characteristic asymmetry, not only in the foot, but, curiously, in the muscles of the leg well above the foot and ankle. Finally, as you might expect, the situation was the same for problems in the shoulder, elbow, lower arm, wrist, hand, and fingers—the presence of visual and non-visual asymmetries of various types. But the pattern of one-sided pain and asymmetry had another element of commonality: the patient's history.

I supplemented the standard patient history questions with detailed questions about the history of patient's physical activities. I wanted to know what the patient had done and was doing during his or her life for work and leisure, including exercise, as well as sleeping and sitting habits, on the then-off chance it might later provide a clue to the process of subluxation or back pain. These supplemental histories began paying me diagnostic dividends. When, for example, a woman came to me complaining of neck and/ or shoulder pain, absent recent trauma, I would almost always find that she was and had been for years a factory worker, secretary, or other category of long-term employee in an occupation requiring hundreds or thousands of repetitive and/or strenuous movements of her arms and hands during her workday. With men, it was the same. Often I would find that men patients who complained of hand, arm, neck, shoulder, or low back pain were usually long-term employees in various types of factory, construction, or other strenuous work involving repetitive tasks and movements.

Similarly, with patients who were not engaged in particularly strenuous or repetitive movement at work, but who were involved in sports or other leisure or hobby activities requiring strenuous, repetitive use of various muscles or muscle groups, I knew where to look for the asymmetry. Eventually, I had identified a number of patterns, whereby patients in certain occupational, leisure, or exercise activities would invariably experience asymmetry, pain, or subluxation in the same areas—usually on one side, or, if on both sides, worse on one side.

Then there were patients who neither worked nor played hard, but who had been in an auto accident, had fallen, or otherwise suffered trauma, strain or sprain—and not necessarily recently. Like the others, once they described what happened, I knew exactly where I would find their asymmetries.

Eventually, regardless of how my patients ended up in my office, once I took their physical activities history and complaints of pain, stiffness, or loss of range of motion, I knew pretty much what type of asymmetry I would find on them. The patterns were clear: If you were one of my patients, all you had to do was tell me what you did and had been doing for a living, what type of leisure activities you pursued and, where necessary, describe your accident, and I could tell you, even before I examined you, exactly where I would find asymmetry.

One day, as a result of my exposure to these patterns, I was hit with my penultimate epiphany on subluxation: subluxation was not in itself a process, but was actually an advanced symptom of another process, which involved increasingly severe and uneven muscle tension, in turn causing joint subluxation, joint pain, back pain, neck pain, general muscle pain and weakness, and asymmetry—even in the absence of pain. So far as I could tell at the time, a major factor in this process was the frequent, repetitive and often strenuous use over time of the muscles involved.

Back then, I didn't have a name for this process, and didn't know what drove it. What I did know was that my comparative palpation and visual exams identified the asymmetry created by this process, and my specialized massage techniques initiated the reversal of the process, beginning with successful manipulation where necessary.

As my with my previous epiphanies, this one begged not one question but several: What started this process, and when, how, and where? Why did this process consistently generate asymmetry on a patient literally from top to bottom? Somehow, I just knew that I was missing an important piece of the puzzle.

By early 1964, a number of changes had taken place in my life. My marriage had ended in divorce and I received custody of my 12-year-old son. Professionally, as my practice became more successful I upgraded my office and living quarters by purchasing a two-story duplex with a full basement at 150 West Mechanic Street in Shelbyville. My son and I lived upstairs, and I relocated my practice to a much roomier office downstairs. Now I had two exam/treatment rooms, a waiting room, a receptionist's office, another small utility room, a bathroom, and my private office. The 13 years I spent on Mechanic Street postured me for my ultimate realization.

After the move to Mechanic Street, I purchased X-ray equipment so I could take, develop, and read my own films. Later I joined the Indiana National Guard Reserves and was commissioned as a Captain. For a time I was also taking the X-rays for the annual physicals of the members of the Guard.

Acquisition of my own equipment gave new meaning for me to the phrase "X-ray vision." As I reviewed thousands of X-rays of regular patients and Guardsmen, three recurrent examples of asymmetry in films of the pelvis attracted my attention. I had seen all three many times in films at Lincoln and in my early practice. Back then, I put them on my "unsolved mysteries" list, but otherwise paid them no particular attention and gave them little further thought.

By the time I moved to Mechanic Street, things were different. These phenomena were three stones unturned, but not for long. One was the puzzling asymmetry in the obturator foramina, the holes in the two ischia, or "butt" bones: one hole was always smaller in diameter than the other whether the X-ray was taken with the patient lying down or standing up. At Lincoln, and probably everywhere else, X-rays of the spine traditionally were taken with the patient lying down. Why, I can't tell you. However, by the time I had developed my new exam procedures and purchased my X-ray equipment, I was taking them with the patient in a standing position. My reasoning was that when a person lies down the

skeleton and supporting musculature are not under stress, so an
X-ray taken in that position literally does not give a true picture of
what's going on. For my diagnostic purposes, X-raying a patient in
a lying position would be like deciding if a new aircraft were flight
worthy without flight testing it. There were two other abnormalities
in the pelvic shots. One was that one ilium, or hip bone, appeared
to be smaller than the other. The other was that one ischium was
lower than the other. Again, why these differences?

I thought about these phenomena frequently, trying to figure
out their significance, but nothing came to me. Were they clues to
the cause of the process that culminates in subluxation? For that
matter, were they cause or effect? It would be a few years before I
would get the answer in the form of my ultimate epiphany.

Eventually as I began to hone my palpation and visual exam
skills more finely, as well as my massage and manipulation techniques, I felt that there was little purpose in keeping my X-ray
equipment, or, for that matter, taking x-rays at all. I could feel spinal
or joint subluxation with my lubricated hands. So, unless my patient
had had an accident after which no X-rays had been taken, I didn't
bother with X-rays any more.

Though I felt that I had removed and improved the only
valuables I could from the field of chiropractic—palpation and
manipulation—I found it necessary to check for a pulse occasionally,
as I was required to attend one or more "continuing chiropractic
education" seminars each year in order to keep my license. Sitting
through these seminars was sheer torture. Besides the title of "D.C."
on my office letterhead and business cards, I felt I had nothing in
common with these other chiropractors. Because the diagnostic and
treatment techniques that had brought me success in my practice
bore little if any similarity to what I'd been taught at Lincoln,
the material I saw presented at these seminars served only to re-
emphasize that in theory and practice, they lived in one world and
I lived in another. As I listened to my colleagues talk about having
trouble with this or that condition or about some new modality
contraption that was supposed to do this or that, it was all I could
do to keep quiet. Yet, I couldn't tell them anything. I was in reality a
very specialized masseur in chiropractor's clothing who was getting

increasingly impressive results with problems that others found difficult or impossible to treat without paying so much as lip service to chiropractic theory or practice. If I tried to explain my own theories and practices, or suggested my belief that the very foundation of chiropractic was flawed, they might label me a heretic or even try to revoke my license. As I did while at Lincoln, I kept silent and continued on my own path toward my ultimate epiphany.

That said, I did dally briefly with a couple of modalities during this period. One was ultrasound. By this time, of course, I was no longer a spring chicken. My massage work, though efficient and effective, was taking a toll on my own body. I wanted to experiment to see if ultrasound—basically low-voltage electrical current used to create mild heat—would loosen up muscles without the need for massage. It didn't, so I discarded it.

By the early to mid-1970's, I'd acquired another modality contraption. It consisted of a small cabinet about the size of a mini refrigerator on wheels. An aluminum pipe with flexible joints protruded from the top of the cabinet. At the top of this pipe was a device which looked like a small bongo drum. For professional use, the idea was to position the drum-like portion so it rested above and faced the area of the patient's body where it was to be used. I honestly can't remember what it was supposed to do. However, whatever it was supposed to do, it apparently didn't impress me, so I got rid of it, too. I will say this about it: it was entertaining. My son loved to demonstrate its non-therapeutic capability for his friends, providing what may have been the first in wireless entertainment. He would turn the device on, pick up a fluorescent light tube, and wave it in front of the drum head. When he did so, the tube lit up and remained illuminated as long as you held it in front of the drum head.

Despite these developments, I was still on a plateau. To be sure, the elevation of this one was much higher than the one I was on when I arrived in Shelbyville. I was successfully treating every musculoskeletal problem that came through the door, literally from head to toe, including one that I had heard that my colleagues couldn't, sciatica. And I didn't confine myself to dealing solely with back, neck, joint, and muscle pain. I had also found the cause of and figured out how to get rid of headaches of all types, including the mother of all headaches, the migraine.

By this time, I had also developed eagle-sharp eyes and incredibly sensitive fingers to locate asymmetries. My focused, specialized massage eliminated my patients' pain, discomfort, stiffness, loss of use, and loss of range of motion. Even if I couldn't completely get rid of the problem with the first visit, I could give them immediate relief. If they took my advice on what to do or not to do in between visits they continued to feel better and were able to see and feel progress after each succeeding visit until they were symptom-free. There was an end to treatment in sight for them. Finally, because I was able to see certain unmistakable, recurrent patterns for many problems, I was now able to tell patients not only where their problems were, but also where they would be having other problems in the future.

For the most part, I was professionally happy. I had turned what I saw as a lemon into the sweetest lemonade. I felt that, given the information made available to me during nearly a quarter century of practice, I had all but perfected my diagnostic and treatment techniques. Yet, even with all that I had accomplished, I still had one more quest: to find the elusive answer to my questions about what caused this so-far-unnamed process that began with asymmetry and pain and ended with subluxation, or worse. . .and what about those asymmetries on the pelvic X-rays? These answers, thankfully, were only a few miles and a few years away.

In the late 1970's, I again combined office and home, this time to a property on the outskirts of Shelbyville, on what was known as Old Michigan Road, or Highway 421 North. On nearly two acres sat a three-bedroom home with attached two-car garage, plus another huge three-door garage that had previously housed tank trucks used in a bulk milk business. I would live and practice here for the about 15 years, experiencing early in that period my ultimate epiphany. . .the one that would answer my remaining questions.

Not long after I relocated my practice to Michigan Road, a man walked into my office complaining of severe leg pain. My exam revealed a number of asymmetries that I had seen many times before. One that especially caught my attention was the fact that the top of one of his hips was much lower than the other. I performed my usual massage technique on a portion of that leg. Within a few minutes, the pain left, and the hip on that leg was slightly higher than the hip on the opposite leg.

Three days later, though, this man returned, along with his complaints of pain in the same leg, again with a lower hip on the painful leg side. This time, I massaged his entire leg on the low hip side. Again, the pain left, and the lower hip again became slightly higher than the hip on the opposite leg. Three days later, he, his leg pain and his lowered hip were back.

By this time, in addition to the patterns I had seen and used in diagnosis, I had also became aware of patterns in the way patients responded to my massage techniques for various problems. In other words, a given patient with a specific problem should be positively responding to my treatment within a certain number of visits. If not, I was either misdiagnosing the problem or there was a problem in addition to the one I had diagnosed. This patient was responding at first but then regressing, suggesting to me that there was another problem.

Our instructors at Lincoln had told us that approximately 11% of the general population had one leg that was shorter than the other, and that this could be responsible for unspecified problems. That was it. We were given no instruction on how to identify this "short leg" or how to treat it. In my practice throughout the years I had yet to see a patient who displayed this short-leg phenomenon, but I was always on the lookout.

While I pondered the unusual response pattern of this patient, I had a flashback. I remembered the three aforementioned skeletal asymmetries I had noticed in the pelvic X-rays over the years: the diameter of one of the obturator foramen smaller than the other, one ilium smaller, and one ischium lower. Then it hit me. Were the lowered hip and rotated pelvis I had found when examining this and other patients the external manifestations of these skeletal asymmetries? If so, were they the reason that the effects of my massage were so short-lived? Was this man my first, long-awaited case of a short leg? There was one way to find out. . .

I decided to experiment. As before, I massaged the whole leg, as well as other areas above the leg, and then I did something else, something I had done with no other patient. I put a lift in his shoe on the painful leg side. Immediately, his hips became level, and within minutes, he started feeling less pain. Three days later, he returned, pain-free. What's more, not only were his hips still level, but there were changes in his pelvis: it was no longer twisted or rotated. Finally, the extraordinary muscle tension in the leg that had been painful was now greatly reduced.

This was my final, long-awaited, and much-needed epiphany. I now had identified and realized how to eliminate the elusive cause of the unequal muscle tension resulting in one-sided low back and sacroiliac pain. I thought about what my instructors at Lincoln had theorized about subluxation, and realized the significance of the three pelvic X-ray abnormalities. The internal stresses—the skeletal abnormalities—were in reality manifested by the external stresses— asymmetries and pain in the musculature of the short leg.

In the months and years that followed, I would see that this "short leg" could and often did cause other problems, not only further down that short leg, but also on the normal leg, and above the hips, too, from head to toe.

CHAPTER 6
The Long and Short of the Short Leg Effect

So far you've seen how, for decades, I'd been trying to discover the inner workings of an unnamed process causing asymmetry, pain and, eventually, spinal and joint subluxation or worse, and usually just on one side. I want to discuss how I came up with a name for this process, why I define it as I do, and the two causes I've found for this phenomenon.

I call the process that took me decades to discover and understand "Musculoskeletal Distortion," or MSD. "Distortion" is the word I believe best describes the asymmetrical, twisted, and disfigured shape your body begins to take as MSD advances.

I define MSD as "The natural, lifelong, and progressive impairment and deterioration of the functioning of the musculoskeletal system." A general description of the symptoms of MSD would include all types of asymmetry in many areas of the body, stiffness, muscle pain, joint pain, loss of use or loss of range of motion in the extremities (among other areas), subluxation, and deterioration in the spine and the joints. MSD appears in many or all areas of your musculoskeletal system, even without your being aware of it. Some will suffer worse symptoms than others, and over more extensive areas, depending on factors I will discuss later.

The easiest way to visualize what I mean by MSD is to look at charts of the muscular system and skeletal system, two of a number of systems in your body. The "musculo" part of the name refers to the many muscles and associated tendons and ligaments that make up most of the muscular system, which, among other things, allows you to move and perform other tasks. The "skeletal" part of the name refers to the system of 200 bones that make up the frame of the adult body. "Musculoskeletal system," then, describes the interactive functioning of these two systems.

"Natural, lifelong, and progressive" refers to the fact that MSD occurs and progresses—gets worse—from nothing more than walking or performing other normal types of movement or work with your legs, feet, hands, fingers, arms, and other parts of the body, and continues to worsen throughout life.

"Impairment and deterioration" occur when the muscular and skeletal systems, both separately and in combination, don't work properly and suffer damage, sometimes permanent.

I have found that MSD has two causes. One is Muscle Overuse, or MO, which I will discuss in the next chapter. The other cause of MSD is what I call the Short Leg Effect, or SLE. In this chapter, I will explain what I mean by the "short leg," how I identify it, and what I mean when I refer to it as an "effect."

From my experiences with patients I have observed a stark difference in the sense in which I think of a short leg and the way at least some other doctors think of a short leg. This difference in thinking is reflected in the different ways we identify the phenomenon. When some doctors say a leg is "short," they mean short in a relative, anatomical sense: that the length of one leg is less than the other leg which, by default, is considered to be of normal length. They attempt to identify the short leg by measuring both legs of the patient, using whatever reference points they deem appropriate, with the patient lying down.

I, on the other hand, have never measured a patient's legs to identify the short leg, for two important reasons. One reason is historical. When I was studying at Lincoln, the issue of whether or not a short leg existed was hotly debated, in part because it was so difficult to identify by measurement. Early on, this debate made me doubt the reliability of measuring. Later, my bias against measuring was only strengthened by treating a number of patients who previously had their short legs misidentified by another doctor through measurement. However, even if I had decided to measure, I would never have done it with the patient lying down. I always examined and X-rayed my patients while they were standing in order to get the true picture of the body functioning under stress.

The second reason is that I see the short leg as a functional short leg, not as an anatomically short leg. In other words, I identify the short leg ultimately by how it performs by using the same method that I successfully used to identify other problem areas: identifying asymmetry through comparison. Asymmetry never lies.

I compare one side of the patient's pelvic area to the other, making a preliminary identification of the short leg from a combination palpation-visual exam, looking for the asymmetry on the outside of the body that I had seen in pelvic X-rays: pelvic rotation and difference in hip height. So reliable is this approach that, unless the patient's history included an accident for which no X-rays had been taken, I don't take X-rays. Because the short leg produces a characteristic gait, I validate my preliminary identification by watching the patient walk a short distance both toward me and away from me. Over the decades, I have found this two-part identification method to be very reliable.

So how do you know if you have a short leg? Based on my experiences in the office and my observations of people outside my office, my answer is that every human being, regardless of age or gender, has a functional short leg. When I say "regardless of age," I mean throughout life, not just in adulthood. Even young children display the characteristic gait of the functional short leg when they begin walking. I estimate from experience that the short leg functionality occurs on the left side about 85% percent of the time.

I don't know what causes the short leg or when it's created, but I have seen some things that make me wonder. One day, many years ago, I was leafing through a book on dissection which featured photos of various portions of dissected cadavers. The photos were offered to illustrate the authors' main point which, ironically if coincidentally, was that the human body is imperfect (asymmetrical, in my lingo) in many areas and ways. Though the authors did not comment on it, I noticed one particular asymmetry in a photo of the femurs, the large bones of the upper legs that are inserted into the hip bones in a ball-and-socket fashion. In that photo, both the neck and the ball-shaped head of one femur were clearly smaller than the other. Thereafter, when I looked at other anatomical charts and drawings, I made a point of comparing femurs, and saw the disparity in every one of them—even in a photo of an X-ray of an Egyptian mummy that was many thousands of years old. I also noticed in these charts and drawings the aforementioned asymmetries in the obturator foramen, ilium, and ischium. What's more, if you look at almost any anatomical chart or drawing, or at an X-ray, you can see the pelvic bone structure and size varies from left to right, and one hip bone appears to be wider and higher.

Assuming that these charts and drawings were produced by artists who looked at either dissected cadavers or X-ray films and simply drew what they saw, these images faithfully reflected these asymmetries. Later, when I obtained my own model of the spinal column and pelvic bones, undoubtedly made from a mold based upon an artist's drawing or sculptor's work, I saw the same differences in the ilium and obturator foramen. These artists couldn't all be wrong, and the arguably universal asymmetries their works revealed were certainly no coincidence. They reproduced what they saw, all from different sources, miles and years apart.

Are the smaller neck and head of one femur a universal trait, as so many anatomical charts and drawings suggest? Does this disparity create or play a role in the functionality of the short leg? Why do children walk with the characteristic gait of the functional short leg even before their bones are fused? Are we born with a functional short leg? Regardless of how these and other questions are eventually, if ever, answered, the fact remains that the functional short leg and its effects are here to stay. For this reason I think it's important to pass on what I've learned about the effect of that functional short leg on the musculoskeletal system.

What I call the "Short Leg Effect" is a specific combination of symptoms of MSD that are caused by the functional short leg. This specific combination of symptoms appears after you begin walking as a child. Over time, these initial symptoms worsen and develop into the more severe symptoms of MSD. For the purpose of this discussion, we will assume the short leg to be the left leg, based on my experience that the left leg is the functional short leg 85% of the time.

One of the first functional short leg problems the body must deal with when a child starts walking is imbalance. Recall that, whether or not one of a child's legs is anatomically shorter, the functional effect is that of a shorter leg. Based on my experience in practice, this functional difference in leg length ranges roughly from one-quarter to one-half inch in most people. Not a great deal of difference, but still enough to cause problems. This imbalance results in a shift of body weight to the left leg. This shift in weight is harmful to the left knee, which must now support more body weight than it normally would. Over time, there often is erosion of the cartilage protecting the ends of the bones comprising the left knee joint, which can ultimately create the need for knee replacement surgery.

In an attempt to restore balance the knee on the right, or normal, leg begins to flex slightly, and remains flexed while you stand, walk, run or perform other activities in an upright position. Unfortunately, while this flexure may improve balance, it means continuous abnormal stress for the pelvic and leg muscles. The body also tries to compensate for this extra "length" on the right by causing the right foot to turn slightly outward to the right with each step. This gradually causes excessive wear on the outside of the heel of the right shoe, usually requiring replacement of the shoes even though the heel of the left shoe may be relatively unworn.

This imbalance also changes the way both of your feet hit the ground when you walk or run. Normally, absent a lift on the left (short leg) side, the heel and sole of that foot strike the ground simultaneously, while the heel of the right foot hits the ground before the rest of the foot. This can change, however, depending on MO in the use of the short leg, the normal leg, or both

A second initial symptom is the gradual, progressive rotation or turning of the left side of the pelvis anteriorly, or toward the front. This rotation will in turn cause the entire torso to rotate, or twist, toward the front as well.

Third, the left hip moves inferiorly and medially, or downward and inward toward the center of the body. This is the "low hip" I've previously mentioned.

Fourth, the left ischium (butt bone), moves lower and stays lower, even when you're sitting, with few exceptions.

Finally, the muscles of the left leg, particularly those of the lower left leg, begin to tighten abnormally, eventually giving the leg the appearance of being smaller, or atrophied. Also, it's not unusual to see a bowed-in effect which, though usually not noticeable or painful, eventually can appear on the inside of the left ankle above the joint. These effects are, to the trained eye, fairly easy to see in person, though they are extremely subtle and develop so gradually that they are usually imperceptible to the individual experiencing them or to casual observers.

To get a partial mental image of what I've described, imagine one of those miniature dime-store skeletons. Remember how it was held together at the joints with little rings so that you could twist and pull the limbs to change the shape of the skeleton? Did you ever notice how the symmetry of the hips and pelvis of the skeleton changed when, for example, you pulled the right foot down while pulling the left hand up? Though exaggerated, that's somewhat how the SLE begins to make you look after you start walking as a child. The problem is not the asymmetry itself but the constant, unnatural, and uneven tension in your musculoskeletal frame that it represents.

This distortion caused by the SLE will only get worse with time and MO. On the left side, extra weight and abnormally taut leg muscles will eventually affect the knee and other joints and musculature of the entire left side in one or more ways, above, in, and below the pelvis. On the right, the consequences of abnormally tight muscles involved in the operation of the knee joint will eventually also spread up into the low back and beyond, as well as down the right leg and beyond.

Because of the way the SLE and MO work together, you will experience more or less severe symptoms of MSD, earlier or later in life, depending on the combined, relative influence of factors I'll discuss in the next chapter.

CHAPTER 7

The MO of Muscle Overuse

Muscle Overuse, or MO, the second of two causes of the symptoms of MSD, is the end result of what I call Accumulated Repetitive Contractions, or ARC. Before I explain what I mean by MO and how it affects muscles, I want to discuss what I mean by ARC and how it progresses into MO.

First, let's talk a bit about the "C" word in ARC, "Contractions," and the system in your body that helps make motion possible through contraction, the muscular system. As I became familiar with MSD and the effects of MO, I realized that, in terms of the capacity of the muscles of the human body to do at least as much harm as good, the muscular system is probably one of the most underestimated systems in the human body. In order to appreciate what I mean by this statement, as well as to understand the role of muscles in creating the symptoms of MSD, it is useful to clarify how muscles and joints work together, and how ARC affects them.

In the muscular system our focus is on contractions, the process by which the muscular system moves us and enables us to perform work through the use of our hands, arms, shoulders, legs, head, torso, and pelvis. Contraction is the action of the muscle shortening itself. Each muscle is composed of many individual muscle fibers, all of which normally contract or shorten in unison. When they do so, they collectively exert a pulling force on a specific area of the body, like bones of an arm or leg, to accomplish work, either in the form of movement of the body, like walking, or varied specific tasks like pulling, pushing, squeezing, reaching, or gripping. Depending on what you want to pull, push, squeeze, reach, or grip, and for how long and how often, these muscle fibers will have to contract more or less forcefully, for a longer or shorter period of time, and more or fewer times.

For example, take the task of bench-pressing weights, accomplished mostly through the triceps muscles on the undersides of our upper arm bones. By contracting these muscles, we are able to push the weights upward. As long as we are able to keep these muscles in a contracted state, we will be able to keep the weights up in the air. When we're ready to lower the weights, we carefully and slowly do so through lengthening or "relaxing" these muscles. The relaxation of a muscle is, of course, the relaxation in unison of the individual muscle fibers.

Thus, whether the work to be performed is bench-pressing, tip-toeing, turning your head, walking, waving, or any of thousands of other movement or work tasks, the process is the same: a single muscle or group of muscles contracts to perform the task, and the work ceases when the muscle or muscle group relaxes.

The skeletal system consists of the vertebrae of the spine; the joints of the body; the bones forming those joints; the ligaments, which attach bones to each other; the tendons, which attach muscles to bones; and the cartilage protecting the ends of the bones from friction generated in the operation of the joints. For example, take the elbow joint, which is formed where the ends of the bones of the lower arm and the upper arm meet at specific angles. This joint allows us to use our upper and lower arms, pulled by the muscles attached to them, to perform various movements and tasks. As with all other joints in the body, cartilage covers the ends of the bones of the joint to prevent friction damage to the bones as the joint operates.

Now let's look at the "R" in ARC, "Repetitive." A repetitive action is one that is repeated over and over again during either a single session or multiple sessions over a given period of time, be it minutes, hours, days, months, years, or decades. Thus, we could be talking about such common activities as walking, pulling, pressing, lifting, gripping, or reaching. But the issue becomes more complicated if you ask not whether you are walking, but how far are you walking, and where? Are you walking uphill, downhill, on sand or snow, and for 1 mile, or 10 miles? What are you pulling, pressing, lifting, or squeezing, and how often? Are you pulling an object off a shelf, or 100 pounds of anti-freeze on a rolling warehouse skid? Are you an elevator operator, or surfing the internet? Are you "working out" on an exercise machine, or lifting 30 pounds of laundry? Are you kneading pizza dough, or playing a video game, and for how long at a stretch? Are you a waitress with a touchpad register, a grocery stock boy or checker? Are you a frequent texter?

Notice that, while these examples encompass a wide variety of typical occupational, leisure, and exercise activities, they all require repeated contraction of particular muscles or muscle groups. Also, note that some of these activities are much more strenuous than others, requiring muscles to work harder per contraction, and to remain contracted for a longer period of time. Finally, remember that the same individual will likely perform at least two or more of these activities, or many other real-life examples we could list, in the same 24-hour period. If these examples don't apply to you, take a moment to mentally list your own daily, weekly, or monthly repetitive activities in the occupational, leisure, and exercise categories. Now it becomes easier to see how repeated contraction contributes to MSD.

Now let's talk about the "A" in "ARC," "Accumulated." Whether you use my examples or yours, now try to imagine performing these daily activities over years or decades. Remember that I'm not talking about just one activity, but the performance of multiple repetitive activities in the same day, many of which use some or most of the same muscles or muscle groups. Thus, it is easy to see that there is an accumulation of repetitive contractions, not just from one activity over time, but from several activities over time.

The ARC of a muscle or muscle group means more than just the long-term history of your total physical activity. It comprises the total number of muscular contractions performed by a muscle or each of the muscles in a muscle group up to a given point in time. It doesn't matter to your muscles whether you classify a given physical activity as work, leisure, or exercise. To your muscles, it's all the same—contraction, contraction, contraction, repeated time after time, daily, weekly, monthly, over years or decades. So, you ask, what's the point? Our bodies are made to last a lifetime, so there's no real limit on the number of contractions a given muscle can perform, right?

Wrong. There IS a limit to the number of contractions for each muscle or muscle group, regardless of the type of motion. Again, muscles don't have separate contraction limits for work, leisure, and exercise activities. When the number of contractions a muscle has performed exceeds that limit, that muscle begins to suffer from Muscle Overuse, MO, which contributes to symptoms of MSD. Over 45 years of trying to figure out not only how to get rid of muscle, back and joint pain, but also what caused it have led me to these conclusions. From examining, diagnosing, and successfully treating thousands, of patients with musculoskeletal problems, literally from head to toe, I was able to see clear patterns in my patients relating various types and locations of asymmetry, muscle pain, joint and back pain, and subluxation to various occupational, leisure, and exercise activities performed by both men and women, over years or decades, that collectively subjected them to MO, and eventually the symptoms of MSD.

What I want to discuss now in general terms is the way in which MO is a contributing cause of MSD. First, the degree to and rate at which the effects of MO cause the symptoms of MSD will vary with the individual, according to his or her ARC. Again, the cold hard fact is that, even with adequate rest, stretching, hydration, and the best of diets, every muscle has a limited number of contractions available to it before it experiences MO. The progression toward MO is much like a timer counting down the minutes to seconds to zero, except that the units counted down are not minutes but available contractions.

What matters is not the chronological age of the muscle subjected to MO—i.e., how old you are—but the accumulated number of contractions the muscle has performed up to a given point in time. The more active you are, the quicker you reach your limit for a given muscle or muscle group. Thus, a more active, much younger man can exhibit the same symptoms of MSD you would expect to see in an older man having performed the same activity.

Let me illustrate my point with a common recreational activity that uses a number of muscles, many of which are also used in other, non-recreational activities: bowling.

I learned from treating bowlers that bowling is a tremendously stressful activity for several areas of the body, adding to the ARC performed by many of the same 100 or so muscles bowlers use to perform other tasks. Let's consider a bowler who is 50 years old and has bowled 2,000 games since age 18, and a bowler who is 35 who has also bowled 2,000 games since age 18. Assume that both have been employed at the same occupation for the same number of years, and work equally hard. Both have roughly the same degree of MSD manifested as low back and shoulder pain. Yet, though both have bowled the same number of games over their lives, the younger man is suffering to the same degree as another man 15 years his senior. Because the younger bowler has bowled the same number of games during a shorter period of time—18 years versus 32 years for the older man—he has surpassed his contraction limits for muscles involved in this activity much earlier in life. All things being equal, if the younger man continues to bowl with the same frequency, he can expect to be in much worse shape by time he reaches 50 than the older man is right now.

At this point it is useful to understand what happens to muscle tissue subjected to MO as well as a few of the more generalized symptoms of MO, such as asymmetry and pain. To begin with, recall that each muscle is composed of many individual muscle fibers. So, again, what we think of as a contraction of the muscle as a whole is really the simultaneous contraction of all muscle fibers in that muscle. When these fibers are not contracted they're relaxed, meaning each of the individual muscle fibers in relaxation has in theory returned to its pre-contraction length. Logic suggests that these muscle fibers can be in only one of two possible physical states: contraction or relaxation.

So, what happens to these muscle fibers when, at some point, they exceed their contraction limits and cross over the line into MO? Well, I'm sure that, on at least one occasion, you have experienced what you might call muscle fatigue from an activity requiring rapid, numerous, and perhaps strenuous contractions of a given muscle or muscle group. Toward the end of your session, your muscle(s) felt weak and didn't contract as quickly or forcefully, causing you to stop the activity for the time being. What you experienced was a glimpse of some of the early, less severe symptoms of MSD that would develop if you were to continue that activity over time.

Though still functional to one degree or another, A muscle affected by MO becomes weak. It can't contract as forcefully or quickly, or as many times during a given period of time, and rest provides less and less of a rejuvenating effect. However since the muscle is still functional, there is only one conclusion to draw: some undetermined but significant number of muscle fibers must be dysfunctional in one of three possible ways: (1) These fibers are fully relaxed, but, for unknown and complex physiological reasons, they can no longer contract; (2) they have become frozen or locked up in a contracted state, unable to relax; (3) these fibers are partially contracted, meaning they still have some percentage of their normal contraction potential available.

My experience with the musculoskeletal system tells me that (2) and (3) are equally plausible explanations for MO weakness. However, in the end, it really doesn't matter whether it's (2) or (3). Why? The reason is that symptoms of MSD are caused in part by taut, shortened muscles. Taut, shortened muscles are in reality taut, shortened muscle fibers, and taut, shortened muscle fibers are contracted muscle fibers regardless of whether "contracted" means partially or wholly contracted. Whichever muscles were involved, when I performed my specialized massage techniques on my patients, their muscles became smoother, longer, and stronger. If my pre- and post-massage muscle testing hadn't already convinced me that MO makes muscles weak, what I learned over the years from treating an especially interesting category of patients would have done so.

I had the good fortune to treat a number of patients who were weightlifters, or body builders, whatever you care to call them. The sight of their heavily-muscled physiques took me back to my youth. My family lived in a rough neighborhood in Buffalo, and instead of hanging out with boys my age who would likely get me into trouble, I joined the Boy Scouts and lifted weights at the YMCA. I, too, developed a heavily-muscled, V-shaped chest. I was even able to put on the classic demonstration of strength, by easily tearing in half with my bare hands the several-inches-thick Buffalo telephone directory.

A weightlifter's body is like an open book illustrating the effects of ARC over a relatively short period of time. Before I began muscle-testing and treating weightlifters, I presumed that hyper-developed muscles would not evidence MO, and would therefore not display the muscle weakness I was accustomed to finding in most patients. However, to my surprise, my muscle testing exposed a number of weaknesses in their upper and lower bodies. Even weightlifters, who you'd expect to be literal pillars of strength, could not escape the muscle-weakening effects of MO achieved through ARC.

I should relate to you one recent example which further validates my assertion that muscles subjected to MO are at least partially dysfunctional and weak. When I performed my specialized massage techniques on my patients, I knew I was initiating reversal of the MO, and hence of MSD. Reversal in essence put more available contractions on the counter, tending to place the involved muscle fibers back under the limit. What I didn't realize for a long time was that my massage was doing something else as well.

Periodically, I performed my specialized massage techniques on a diabetic friend to ease symptoms of MSD. On one particular occasion, my friend tested her blood sugar before and after the massage session. I had decades earlier experimented by taking pre- and post-massage blood pressure readings on my patients. I

found that post-massage BP was always lower, clearly due, in my
opinion, to the reduction of the tautness in the massaged muscles,
allowing blood to flow into and out of the muscle with less effort.
This phenomenon was consistent with the fact that blood pressure is
often higher when taken on one arm versus the other. This would be
explained by the fact that the arm with the higher reading was either
the dominant arm, or was in any event subjected to ARC from one
or more activities.

Thus, I was not surprised when my friend's post-massage blood
sugar tested 100 points lower after my massage. I could think of
only two possible explanations for this drop. One would be that,
as with BP, less blood flow—and therefore less blood sugar—was
made available to my friend's contracted, dysfunctional muscles,
and reversal of the dysfunctionality by massage allowed more blood
flow. The other possibility was that, to whatever degree, because
my friend's muscles were in a dormant-like state of dysfunctionality
before the massage, they utilized much less sugar from the blood
that did reach them. Again, reversal of their dysfunctionality
through massage enabled them to use more sugar.

As MO of an already dysfunctional muscle becomes severe, the
degree of the dysfunctionality increases, expressed on the micro level
as an increase in the number of partially or totally contracted muscle
fibers, and on the macro level by a muscle that gets shorter and
tighter. As it does so, additional or more pronounced asymmetry
appears in the form of inflammation of the muscle tissue, which can
be felt through the skin. Also, as the muscle gets shorter and tighter,
it loses its smooth texture in one or more places along its length.
This loss of smoothness will show up as various forms and sizes of
uneven or raised areas in the body of the muscle that can also be
felt through the skin and that may be painful when varying degrees
of pressure is applied to them. If it has not already, this muscle
tissue will, at some point, display additional classic asymmetry by
appearing to be either flatter or rounder than its counterpart muscle
on the other side of the body. Some of these symptoms will also
appear in a portion of the muscle closer to a joint. Muscle spasms
may occur, too, lasting from a few seconds to several minutes or

longer, and may return several times during the day or over a period of days. Last, but certainly not least, there is pain in the muscle, with or without use of the muscle, especially those muscles in the lower back, shoulder, between the shoulder blades, in the chest, legs, buttocks, neck, jaw, extremities, and joints. This pain may be mild at first, and for a while may come and go.

These, then, are some of the early, less severe symptoms of MSD resulting from MO. Though the process of muscular dysfunction seems logical and straightforward, based on my years of experience treating MSD I would like to dispel what I see as a number of myths believed by most people about how the musculoskeletal system works:

Myth #1: The site of the pain is the cause of the pain.

I have found this common belief to be incorrect. In fact, my cardinal diagnostic rule is that the site of the (MSD) pain is not the cause of the pain. When you experience pain in muscles or a joint, you are subconsciously programmed to think that the cause of the pain is located in the same spot as the pain itself. In the case of a bee sting, for example, you'd be right: the stinger at the pain site is the cause of the pain. However, in the case of an MSD pain site, you'd be wrong. My decades-long experience with reversing MSD has taught me that what's causing the pain is not only located elsewhere, but is sometimes so far away from the pain site that you might not believe it. Take for example, pain on the bottom of the foot, with or without heel pain. As I will later explain to you, this problem is really a symptom of MSD, and its cause lies elsewhere, well above the foot.

Myth #2: Exercise strengthens muscles.

Again, not true. A larger muscle is composed of larger individual muscle fibers, which, collectively, make it stronger. But, as we saw from the earlier discussion about weightlifters, even athletes' strong muscles are not immune to the effects of ARC, and will become weak with numerous "reps." If anything, exercise—again just another activity label for muscular contraction—will contribute, along with work, and leisure (sports activities included) to ARC, which will transition to MO, which in turn contributes to the development of the symptoms of MSD.

In the context of MO, it's important to clarify what is meant by "exercise." Most people would define exercise as activities such as running, walking, playing tennis, aerobics, weightlifting, or working through a room full of high tech "workout" machines. That's fine, but, since all of these activities are accomplished by ARC, how are any of these distinguishable from other activities requiring the use of muscles, except, perhaps, by the frequency, level of intensity, duration, or number of repetitions? Remember, your muscles do not distinguish between contractions done for work, leisure, or exercise. However these activities are classified, muscles perform work by contracting.

When you hit the gym, tennis court, or biking trail after you're finished working for the day, you of course don't think about these activities as examples of ARC. You see the pursuit of these activities as a switch from one activity to another, from work to leisure, exercise, or sports, as if switching from one computer software application to another, or from one DVD to another. Unfortunately, when you switch activities, you don't switch musculoskeletal systems.

My intent is not to pass judgment on the claimed cardiovascular or other benefits of exercise. I am here to say that, depending upon your ARC from other physical activities, exercise may have its price which, for many, will be one or more of the group of severe symptoms of MSD that we will discuss later. The bottom line is that you only have so many total contractions available to you before you start having problems—the symptoms of MSD—so it's really a matter of figuring out where you spend your limited contractions. Remember my weightlifter patients? If exercise is supposed to strengthen the muscles, what happened in their case?

Let me run by you another illustrative "exercise" anecdote from my experience in practice. Beginning in the 1980's, many people, women in particular, were caught up in the aerobics craze. It was hailed, particularly by those who stood to gain financially, as the perfect way to burn fat, tone muscles, "sculpt" the body, and attain cardiovascular fitness. If you ever participated in such a class or watched an aerobics video, what did you experience or see? Anywhere from 30 minutes to an hour of fast-paced ARC involving many muscle groups. As time has proven, whether it was or wasn't the perfect way to attain what was seen as fitness, it was the perfect way to achieve or advance something else: the severe symptoms of MSD. How do I know? This kind of exercise, often in addition to dancing, biking, running, and other activities, was in the physical activities histories of numerous women patients in my office in that era complaining of pains in the knees, arms, chest, elbows, feet, and legs—even sciatica. While I stand firm on my statement that the symptoms of MSD are not age-related, I would have expected to see these symptoms of MSD in much older women. What I saw in the office made it clear to me that the MO resulting from the exercises these women pursued were clearly responsible for the advanced symptoms of MSD they suffered.

Myth #3: Back pain is caused by weak muscles.

Wrong again. By now it's probably clear why I list this as a myth. Back pain is a symptom of MSD and is caused by MO and the SLE. As I've explained, ARC will over time create weak muscles, and exercise is but one potential contributor to MO. Over the years, I have met countless people—patients and non-patients alike—who literally suffer because of this popular misconception about back pain. They see that when they move around, their back pain stops. From this, they conclude that they are getting rid of their back pain because this exercise strengthens their weak back muscles. Of little notice to them is the fact that later, after they stop moving around, their back pain returns, often worse than before. So why does their pain subside when they get up and move? What is happening is a phenomenon that has to do in part with what occurs when ARC has crossed over the line into MO.

I have found that, inexplicably, and especially with back pain, after MO reaches a certain point, muscles begin to lose their sensitivity to pain. Either the pain threshold rises or, as a protective mechanism, muscles further affected by MO lose the ability to register pain during use, but upon rest regain the ability to register pain. This phenomenon may be related to yet another pain phenomenon that I observed in my patients.

As I grew increasingly effective with my specialized massage technique over the years, I became curious about an item of post-massage feedback from my patients. Although they felt better in many ways the day of or after I had massaged their problem area(s), they temporarily, for 24 to 48 hours, experienced generalized pain over many of the areas of I had massaged. The pattern that emerged here was that the severity of the pain they experienced was proportional to both the degree of pressure I had applied in the massage and the duration of the massage in a given area. What's more, for patients whose course of treatment required multiple sessions, this mysterious pain was less and less severe with each subsequent visit or, in some cases, occurred only after the first visit. This phenomenon was so predictable that I eventually warned my patients that they might later, either that day or the next, feel "like they'd been hit by a truck," but that they should not worry—it was natural and temporary. Here again, since what my massage was doing was initiating reversal of the MSD by relaxing and lengthening, and therefore strengthening, the affected muscles, I could only conclude that somehow, on the one hand, as the muscle fibers begin to become dysfunctional they lose the ability to register pain, yet, on the other hand, as they "reawaken" and regain lost functionality, they regain the ability to be painful. While this unexplained "pain in, pain out" phenomenon is certainly interesting, my point here is that neither exercise nor any other kind of contraction-based activity strengthens these weak muscles, but only serves to make them even more dysfunctional. The temporary cessation of pain associated with exercising already weak and painful muscles in the back is, in my opinion, a purely self-protective phenomenon.

Myth #4: "Sit up straight, with your shoulders back, or you'll get bad posture."

Do you remember when your parents used to tell you that, especially at meals? However well-intentioned, I have found this to be a useless piece of advice, based upon a generalized misunderstanding of what causes an individual's posture. As we will see later, your posture is determined by your physical activities, not by how you sit. Bad posture is a common symptom of MSD, caused mostly by MO.

Myth #5: Heat is good for painful muscles.

Again, applying heat, whether in the form of a heating pad or submersion in hot water, is the worst thing you can do to painful, stiff muscles, which are somewhat inflamed already. Heat causes the muscle tissue to further engorge with blood in order to cool off the tissue heated by the water. This will further aggravate the already shortened, contracted muscle, and make the situation worse. Proper application of ice water packs to these tissues, not heat, reduces inflammation and swelling.

Myth #6: Stiffness is an inevitable part of old age.

This is nonsense. Stiffness, which is another way of referring to taut, dysfunctional muscles leading to decreased joint function, is yet another symptom of MSD, caused by MO. The simultaneous occurrence of stiffness and older age is purely coincidental. Let me offer one of many examples from my decades of practice: I once had an octogenarian woman patient who had been "stiff" for years, and could barely walk the first time I saw her. When I was finished treating her, she was able to take up ballroom dancing. How would this be possible if her stiffness were a consequence of her age? My treatment did nothing to change her age, obviously, yet it enabled her to regain movement she had lacked for many years.

Myth #7: Osteoarthritis is a "condition" or illness in and of itself.

Nothing could further from the truth, as I have come to know and eliminate this severe symptom of MSD. Yes, osteoarthritis is a symptom. . .a symptom of advanced MSD, which, again, is the result of the SLE and MO. Let me explain.

"Osteoarthritis" means inflammation of a bone joint. Conventional healthcare looks at this bone joint inflammation as an illness, disease, or condition in and of itself, and claims that it results from gradual wear and tear or trauma on the joint, which first destroys the cartilage protecting the ends of the bones, and eventually the bare ends of the bones as they rub against one another. Conventional healthcare deals with the pain, stiffness, swelling, inflammation, and lost range of motion with drugs such as narcotics or NSAIDS, or invasive joint replacement/fusion surgery, depending on the severity of these symptoms and whether they occur in the larger joints like the knee or hip, or the smaller joints such as the wrist, elbow, or ankle. Physical therapy is sometimes prescribed to increase the range of motion in the joint, or strengthen the muscles involved.

Before I give you my thoughts on osteoarthritis, I should explain what I mean by "conventional" healthcare. Most of the time I use this term to refer in the aggregate to those U.S. medical doctors who—to the extent they attempt it at all—strive to eliminate the symptoms of MSD I list in this book with drugs, other chemicals, or surgery. I define "conventional" in this way in order to provide a basis for comparison between how the ostensible majority of medical doctors in the U.S. look at and eliminate these symptoms, versus the way in which I look at and eliminate them. Of course I realize that other U.S. healthcare providers, particularly chiropractors, also attempt to eliminate some of these same symptoms of MSD. My distinction, however, focuses on those providers who address the problem with drugs, chemicals or surgery, and for those chiropractors who follow this course, I would consider them also to be part of "conventional" healthcare.

In my practice, I came to know and approach the elimination of osteoarthritis differently than practitioners of conventional healthcare. I reasoned that, over time, the SLE and MO in the musculature involved in a joint, whether a knee or a finger joint, cause an unrelenting, ever-increasing pull on the joint, causing subluxation and/or a decrease in the normal joint spacing. The cartilage-covered ends of the bones are pulled into misalignment and begin rubbing against one another. This unnatural rubbing turns normally gradual wear into destructive, accelerated wear, eventually producing the aforementioned symptoms of osteoarthritis, which is, as I see it, an advanced symptom of MSD.

To treat osteoarthritis, as with other symptoms of MSD, I first apply specialized reversal massage to the taut musculature involved with the joint. Then, where possible, I manipulated the joint back into place, thereby restoring the normal joint spacing and ending the erosion produced by the ends of the bones rubbing together. The results have been the same as with my first successful knee manipulation: the pain, swelling, subluxation, inflammation, and other symptoms disappeared, because I eliminated what really caused the osteoarthritis.

A patient who experiences a fracture will often feel pain around the fracture site after the healing period has passed. Conventional healthcare will associate this pain with the fracture and diagnose it, too, as osteoarthritis. To the contrary, I believe that what the patient is experiencing is muscle pain. As I came to visualize the situation in my practice, the trauma causing the fracture affected not just the bone, but the involved musculature. Additionally, it's likely the patient was displaying some degree of MSD in that musculature before the trauma. Unlike many practitioners of conventional healthcare, I see the need to treat the musculature also. I had a number of fracture patients in my office who experienced this post-healing pain near the fracture site and were told by conventional healthcare that they had osteoarthritis. After I massaged the affected musculature, this "osteoarthritis" disappeared.

Myth #8: Subluxation is limited to the spine.

This is absolutely false. Recalling my first knee manipulation, you probably saw this one coming. The subluxation, or shifting, of the bones of a given joint from their normal angle or position relative to one another is caused by the uneven pulling force of dysfunctional muscles on the ligaments attaching the bones to one another and tendons attaching the muscle to the bone in that joint. The joint space—the space between the ends of the bones—will either increase, potentially signaling a future joint separation, or decrease, causing the ends of the bones to rub together, preceding the onset of osteoarthritis. Especially in the case of the knee, the most complex and most unstable joint in the body, it's possible for joint space to decrease in one area and increase in another. Subluxation is silent, gradual and, at first, painless, as the bones don't register pain while they begin to shift from their normal positions or angles. However, as the increase or decrease in joint space from subluxation heads toward separation or erosion, the tug of war among taut muscles, ligaments, and tendons produces the pain, inflammation, and swelling of osteoarthritis.

In my practice, I have successfully massaged back to relaxation and manipulated back to normality just about every joint literally from head to toe. I can't tell you how many times I took in a new patient who had been told by conventional healthcare that the pain in his or her knee, elbow, wrist, finger, toe, ankle, foot, hip, shoulder, or vertebra was osteoarthritis, and then eliminated that pain, inflammation, swelling and loss of use or range of motion by reversing the subluxation with massage and manipulation. Eventually, when the SLE and MO advance to a certain point, something has to give, and it's usually the joint, whether in the form of subluxation leading to erosion or separation.

CHAPTER 8
How SLE Plus MO Equals MSD

Over the last three chapters I've explained my concepts of Musculoskeletal Distortion, the Short Leg Effect, Accumulated Repetitive Contractions, and Muscle Overuse. In Chapters 9 through 14, I'll identify the specific symptoms of MSD caused by the synergy of the SLE and MO. In this chapter, however, I want to give you a bit more detail about how SLE and MO work together to cause the severe symptoms of MSD.

Having, I hope, dispelled a few myths about how the musculoskeletal system operates as I came to know it over 45 years of practice, I would now like to talk about some non-mythical concepts, beginning with the role of Muscle Overuse in causing the more severe symptoms of Musculoskeletal Distortion. As you'll recall, I've stated that the extent to which and severity of which a given individual shows the symptoms of MSD at a given point in time tends to be proportional to that individual's MO. From the example of the two bowlers, you recall that you display this or that symptom of MSD because of what you've done with your body, how much, how often, and how intensely, not because of how old you are. As you also learned, every time you use a muscle or muscle group, the number of available "under-the-limit" contractions is reduced, regardless of how you categorize your activity. There are no separate limits for muscular contractions used at work, play, or exercise—they all count down the same.

Thus, on one hand, it is possible that someone who has not worked or exercised to any significant degree may die having escaped the severe symptoms of MSD. On the other hand, someone who has combined decades of hard work, strenuous recreation activities, and regular exercise is far more likely to suffer some of the more severe symptoms of MSD. While each of the individuals at and between these extremes of lifetime activity has a functional short leg, it is the individual who was physically active at work, recreation, and exercise who is far more likely to experience the surgery and disability that go with the more severe symptoms of MSD. Career athletes, especially those at the professional level who weight-train, are probably at the greatest risk for the most severe symptoms of MSD, particularly knee problems.

You now know that the apparently universal existence of the functional short leg begins with musculoskeletal impairment and deterioration from the moment we begin walking as children. You also know that MO generally increases one's potential for developing the severe symptoms of MSD. Accordingly, it becomes easy to see the role of the SLE for what it is: a predisposition to the more advanced symptoms of MSD, just as a person can be predisposed to heart failure by family history. Since such a predisposition is only a potentiality, the person with a family tree full of bad hearts can effectively avoid heart problems suffered by other family members, all things being equal, with strict attention to diet. Similarly, then, the role of the SLE is a predisposition we each have to the severe symptoms of MSD.

But MO is not the only factor that determines whether or not we'll develop severe symptoms of MSD. Another variable that we also can control is something which, even with considerable MO, slows the progression of the SLE and therefore the onset of the severe symptoms of MSD for at least several crucial joints. That variable is the shoe lift on the short leg side. My anecdotal description of what it did for my first functional short leg patient might give you an idea how important the lift is, but, unless you've had severe symptoms of MSD in your back, legs and feet, only to feel them disappear almost overnight after you begin wearing a lift in the shoe on the foot of the functional short leg—or having your functional short leg side shoe built up—you can't really appreciate how crucial that lift really is in the overall effort to slow the progression of the SLE, MO notwithstanding. Contrary to the philosophy of many healthcare professionals, I firmly believe that the lift must be worn at all times the patient is on his or her feet, regardless of the nature of the physical activity or the style of footwear. I do not believe that the body should be relied upon to eventually rid itself of the functional short leg. In fact, I contend that the body can't get rid of the SLE at all. The lift slows the progression of the SLE and provides a counterpoint to the effects of the SLE, but the SLE is an effect that is here to stay and thus must be approached as something to be managed rather than eliminated.

That's not to say, however, that there won't be a significant number of people who make it through life—or almost through life—without a lift, and do just fine. These people are those whose lifetime MO is minimal, because their ARCs are below average in number. Because of their relative inactivity, progression of the SLE and therefore development of the severe symptoms of MSD is slowed. They will likely experience only the more transparent, painless symptoms of MSD for many years. Nevertheless, it is quite possible that, later in life, they may still have to undergo knee or hip replacement, for example, due to the delayed onset of MSD. They will never connect the erosion of a joint to MO and the SLE.

The last variable, which is also completely controllable, is nothing short of amazing because it initiates reversal of MSD. The variable is my reversal massage technique, based on phenomena reflecting two operating principles of the musculoskeletal system as it reacts to MO. Every one of the symptoms I'll discuss in later chapters has responded to a combination of my specialized reversal massage technique and the use of a shoe lift on the short leg side. This treatment effectively eliminates pain, swelling, and asymmetry, and, in many cases, makes surgery unnecessary. What's more, my reversal massage has helped my patients regain lost range of motion and use—in effect, putting additional available muscle contractions on the counter, regardless of age.

As you can see, the likelihood that you'll experience the more severe symptoms of MSD depends on the degree to which your SLE is amplified and advanced by MO, minus the effects of a short-leg-side shoe lift and reversal massage. That is not to say that rest and stretching don't play a role. However, once you've subjected a given muscle or muscle group to MO, rest has less and less effect. Some of the pain and stiffness may subside with rest, but these symptoms don't take long to return since you will still maintain a baseline degree of MO. And, as a practical matter, how much can the average person really rest his or her muscles? You can cut out most leisure and exercise activities, but many of the muscle contractions needed for leisure and exercise are also needed for work and other everyday activities.

Likewise, I have found that, as MO intensifies and the severe symptoms of MSD begin to appear, stretching is less and less effective and can even be counterproductive. Stretching is more effective when used before significant buildup of ARCs—the earlier in life, the better. At this point, only reversal massage will effectively eliminate these symptoms. Many of my patients suffering from a variety of the severe symptoms of MSD who, having had the benefit of my massage, were able to achieve a net reversal of MSD, even while continuing to work. Think of trying to bail water out of a sinking boat while water is still leaking in through a hole in the bottom—it's possible, but it will take a little longer.

So how does Muscle Overuse enable the Short Leg Effect to realize its full potential for causing the more severe symptoms of Musculoskeletal Distortion? Let's recap what MO has to work with by recalling the developing distortion of your frame that began with your first steps in childhood. On the left side, you had extra weight on your knee, and your hip has begun to rotate forward, inward, and down. On your right side, the musculature of your knee joint was stressed with every step you took as the body attempts to re-balance you by keeping that knee in a slightly flexed or bent position. Thus, you're starting out in life with a twisted frame that, without help from MO, has already created unequal muscle tension between the left and right sides of the body. You wouldn't notice these initial symptoms of MSD, but it doesn't take a mechanical engineer to figure out that, if you were a robot on the assembly line, you'd never make it past quality control inspection. But since you're not a robot and can't be rebuilt, you'll have to deal with the impact MO will have on your SLE for a lifetime.

With that description in mind, let's fast-forward from the day you take your first steps as a child to some point later in your life—it could be later in childhood, your teens, twenties, thirties or later. The age is not important—what matters is the fact that MO can develop at any time in life. For the purposes of this example, let's say you are in your mid-thirties. If you've been relatively inactive in work, play, or exercise, you haven't developed much ARC and therefore you have little or no MO. Thus, you've probably experienced only a few of the earlier, less severe symptoms of MSD.

If, however, your level of activity has been average to significantly above average or greater, your ARC has imperceptibly transitioned into MO and has advanced your SLE to the point where you have begun to experience a few symptoms of MSD: periodic pain in various muscles and joint pain in the extremities, back, neck, shoulder, or hip, more often than not on the right side. You may also experience occasional or frequent pain of short or long duration in the hands or feet, in the pelvic area, and in the knees, ankles, calves, or elbows. If your MO has significantly advanced, you may have already experienced some of the severe symptoms of MSD, including severe pain in and compromised use of the knee, elbow, shoulder, back, foot, hand, or other joints; torn ligaments or tendons; or some sort of disability. You may have already had or are contemplating surgery for one or more of these problems. Again, the odds are that these problems have occurred on the right side, but they can appear on either or both sides of the body, depending on the influence of ARC and MO in other areas of the body.

So how does Muscle Overuse advance the progression of the Short Leg Effect into more severe symptoms of Musculoskeletal

Distortion? MO does so by taking advantage of phenomena that are reflective of three operating principles of the musculoskeletal system. The first operating principle you already know: MO creates muscles that are taut because the muscle fibers are frozen or locked up in a contracted state.

The way that muscles in such a contracted, taut state react to certain situations is illustrative of a second operating principle of the musculoskeletal system. Besides being dysfunctional, these taut, contracted muscles are also relatively inflexible. When a pulling force is exerted on a taut muscle by other muscles, rather than stretch, the taut muscle tends to pull on other muscles either directly, or indirectly through a joint. This second set of muscles, especially if likewise taut, will in turn pull on a third set of muscles, and so on. This "chain-reactional pulling" can extend from one end or one side of the body to another—and not necessarily in a straight line—until the original pulling force is felt in a muscle, muscle group, or part of an extremity far removed from the muscle or muscle groups which initiated the pulling.

This ability of the musculoskeletal system to export the effects of taut, inflexible musculature from one part of the body to create the more severe symptoms of MSD in another part of the body by chain-reactional pulling illustrates a third musculoskeletal operating principle: all muscles in the body are connected to each another, directly or indirectly. Let me give you three real-life examples of this principle in action.

Many years ago, while moving backward during a racquetball rally, my son came down on his left big toe, bending it back at an angle of ninety degrees or more. Several days later, after the initial pain and discomfort in that foot had disappeared, he began to experience pain and discomfort in the left leg calf, then in the left thigh, and in turn the left buttock, and then partially down the back of the right thigh.

Another example is the case of a woman patient of mine who suffered a freakish, severe sprain on the inside of her left ankle. Initially, the pain was confined to her left ankle joint and foot, but within three or four days, the pain had migrated up the side of the left calf, and later into the inside of the left thigh.

The third example is unfortunately familiar to many readers: "whiplash." Usually the result of auto accidents, and much more violent and painful than the other two examples, whiplash also triggers this same chain-reactional pulling, usually involving muscles in the back, neck, or both. As with the first two examples, the ultimate effect of this chain-reactional pulling may not be felt for days or longer after the impact since the muscles take time to react. This could be the case because the event could be considered a chain-reactional pulling of muscle fibers, some of which are locked into contraction. Severity of the impact aside, the fact that one person's whiplash injury is significantly more painful than another's is, in my experience, due to the fact that since one individual's back, neck, and shoulder musculature may already affected by severe MO, most if not all of the muscles involved are somewhat taut to begin with, compared to the muscles of another person experiencing less severe whiplash whose muscles are far less affected by MO. What really happens in whiplash is that relatively asymptomatic, moderate MSD becomes symptomatic, aggravated by the violent pulling of the muscles in response to the impact. Just as whiplash is different from the other two examples in terms of the violence of the initial pull, it is correspondingly different in terms of the proportionately more severe response the chain-reactional pulling provokes.

Except in terms of intensity of the initial pull, the effect of whiplash is no different than what happens when you attempt to pull or stretch a muscle that's already taut: the muscle is going to react by getting even tauter and pulling back even more forcefully. It's as if the muscle is saying, "The harder you pull me, the harder I'm going to pull back." Therefore, it is better to massage the muscle than to pull at it. Fortunately for some whiplash patients in my practice, I was able to get my hands on them the day of or immediately following the impact and cut short the chain-reactional pulling and accompanying pain with reversal massage, thereby negating the effect of the impact.

In my experience, with one exception, the end results of MO-based chain-reactional pulling—the severe symptoms of MSD—are felt long after the MO which helped produced them. This is because the development of taut, inflexible muscles is more gradual, and so is the chain-reactional pulling. As I began to appreciate these two operating principles, I developed my cardinal diagnostic rule:

The SITE of the pain is NOT the CAUSE of the pain.

With heel pain, for example, I realized the root cause of this pain, MO, lies outside the foot, far up the leg and beyond. The pain in the heel is but one of many symptoms of MSD that I will likely find as I trace the heel pain to its root cause or source. It's the same with pain in the hand, which also is actually the end of the contraction chain reaction induced by MO. As with the heel pain, the root cause is not in the hand, but elsewhere up the arm and beyond, so I will surely find additional MO-based tautness, dysfunctionality and more or less severe symptoms of MSD in other areas, too.

Some chain-reactional pulling due to MO, as in the case of the heel and the hand, starts higher up in a given limb and moves downward to exert its most severe effect on the extremity because this pulling has reached the last link in the chain. However, because of the SLE on the legs, the chain reactional pulling can also move upward from the legs, through the pelvis, up into the lower back or, as you will read later, from the shoulders up into the neck and head. Chain-reactional pulling, then, is a two-way street. In the end, though, whether the chain-reactional pulling moves down the limbs or upward through the torso, the result is the same: Symptoms of MSD in one end of the body are the result of the reaction to the impact of MO upon muscles in another part of the body, accomplished through chain-reactional pulling which takes advantage of the principle that all muscles are connected.

As you may now understand, this across-the-body chain-reactional pulling is the chief reason that stretching is less and less effective as MSD progresses because the muscle you attempt to stretch is not the only muscle affected by MO. When you attempt to stretch a muscle, the resistance you meet is not just from the muscle you're attempting to stretch or pull, but also from many other taut muscles that are "connected" to that muscle over the path of the chain-reactional pulling. Effective stretching is also thereby thwarted when, as is often the case, the path of the chain-reactional pulling on the muscle you're trying to stretch is not a straight line.

As I mentioned earlier, there is one exception to the general rule that the effects of chain-reactional pulling at work in the progression of MSD are delayed. The exception is a result of the chain-reactional pulling that occurs when you sit, especially for long periods of time. When you sit, the effects of the chain-reactional pulling from the SLE and MO can be felt much sooner. The reason is that sitting, especially for long periods, accelerates the rate of the chain-reactional pulling. Why? To answer that question, let's take a look at what happens to two key areas of your musculature when you sit.

Though you'd seldom think about it, when you sit down, the straight line your body formed when you were standing approximates two ninety-degree, or right, angles: one at the waist and the other at the knees. Even for a person who displays only the milder asymmetry and muscle tautness from the SLE and MO, the formation of these right angles upon sitting has negative consequences. The right angle at your waist causes additional pulling of the muscles in the front and in the back in the thighs, hips, pelvis, and abdominal areas, which are already taut and relatively inflexible. Likewise, the muscles involved in the knees, already taut from MO, are now further affected by additional chain-reactional pulling from the tops and sides of the thighs.

The additional pulling aggravates the already taut muscles, resulting in stiffness and/or pain. As a consequence of the right angle formed at the waist, a person can and often does experience stiffness and/or pain in the low back, as well as stiffness in the buttocks and hips upon rising. Also, while sitting one can and often does feel stiffness and/or pain in the side and/or top of one or both knees.

The aforementioned scenario assumes, of course, that the angle formed at the waist is approximately ninety degrees. Unfortunately, for reasons known only to chair manufacturers, most chairs slope downward at the point where the seat meets the backrest so, in actuality, the interior angle formed at the waist becomes less than ninety degrees while the exterior angle, which is where the muscles are being pulled, increases. This creation of obtuse angulation (an angle greater than ninety degrees) further increases the harmful stretching, with proportionately greater potential for stiffness and/or pain. The worst-case scenario, in my experience, is sitting in a recliner, which can increase these angles even further by almost folding you in half at the waist in the sitting position. Recliners, especially those with heavy padding on the headrest, are also bad news for the cervical spine. When you recline, even if only partially, the resistance of the headrest padding uses the weight of your head to apply a continual but super-slow motion version of whiplash to your cervical spine by pushing your head forward, as though you were leaning against a wall with your head or as though someone were standing behind you and pushing your head forward. The stretching effect created by this continual pushing aggravates the muscles in the back of the neck, starting a chain-reactional pull that goes up the back of the head and often continues over the top of the head and down into the forehead, potentially producing a severe headache in that area and/or in the back of the head.

The thickness of the padding in a chair or couch is important, too. My initial scenario also assumed that the seat of the chair is not well-padded. In a plush chair or a couch with cushions that let you "sink," not only are you subjected to extra chain-reactional pulling, but the risk for stiffness and/or pain in the lower back is increased, as the ischium, or butt bone, on the short leg side continues to be lower, aggravating the existing SLE in the pelvic area. Also, as with the recliner, the angle at the waist is exaggerated, so the amount of pull from this extra stretching is increased.

With the knees, the situation is the same. If your knees already suffer from some of the symptoms of MSD, your discomfort will be made worse when you sit, especially if you sit with your lower legs folded underneath your chair as opposed to extending straight to the floor from your knees. If the tension in the knees, especially just above the kneecaps, is especially severe, injury to the knee can result from sitting on the floor with your knees underneath you, or from a movement as simple as kneeling on one knee. The severe, yet often painless tension waits in ambush for just that last bit of tension supplied by the severe pulling that results from the flexing of the knee during the otherwise natural act of kneeling on one knee. One case comes to mind in which an individual with severe pre-existing knee tension in both knees tore a knee ligament merely by kneeling, on one knee, on the mattress of the bed while reaching across the bed to retrieve an object. Sometimes when your knee tension is only moderate, if you kneel on one or both knees in such a fashion as to fold your legs underneath you, you may hear and feel a spontaneous auto-manipulation in the center of one or both knees. The knees were already subluxated, but you wouldn't know it until you accidentally self-manipulate them back into place. This individual was not so lucky.

CHAPTER 9

The March of MSD:
The Pelvic Subsystem

In previous chapters I explained my conceptions of ARC, MO, the SLE, MSD and the relationships between them. In this chapter I will begin to identify the severe symptoms of MSD that I believe are caused by the SLE and MO in differing proportions in different areas of the body. However, first let me clarify how I define a few terms.

First, I have used and will continue to use the word "symptom" to describe a musculoskeletal problem I've identified as being caused by MSD. My use of the word "symptom" in this context reveals a crucial difference between the way conventional healthcare looks at musculoskeletal problems and the way I do. Many of the problems I describe as symptoms are viewed and treated by mainstream healthcare as specific illnesses or ailments, or, more commonly, "conditions" in their own right. While it is not my intention to engage in a debate about whether a given musculoskeletal problem is a "symptom," or a "condition" in its own right, I do want to emphasize that, in my practice, I have found that all of the musculoskeletal problems I mention are symptoms of MSD, which I found to be caused by the SLE and MO.

I have always believed that, whenever possible, treatments should address the cause of a problem, not the symptoms. Why?

Because how you classify a problem—as a "condition" or a symptom—makes a big difference in how you deal with it, and, more importantly, how successful you are in dealing with it. Do firefighters aim their hoses at the smoke, or the fire? Moreover, as you know, when you eliminate one symptom with a drug, you can and often do create one or more other symptoms, some of which are worse than the symptoms for which you resorted to drugs in the first place. Likewise with resorting to surgery to remove symptoms, you usually end up developing additional symptoms related to the surgical procedure—and the cause remains. In my practice, I have eliminated the cause of what I call symptoms of MSD—the progression of the SLE, amplified by MO—with reversal massage and a shoe lift, while conventional healthcare can only attempt to eliminate or reduce temporarily the severity of what are called "conditions" with drugs or surgery.

Second, before I define "pelvic subsystem," I want to clarify what I mean by "subsystem." Over the years, through detailed patient activity histories, I began to see the patterned relationships between ARC, MO, the SLE, and the types and locations of the symptoms of MSD displayed by my patients. As a result, I came to visualize and analyze the dysfunctionality of the musculoskeletal system in a different way based on my cardinal diagnostic rule: The site of the pain is not the cause of the pain. As I became more familiar with how MSD comes about and progresses, instead of looking at the musculoskeletal system as a one gigantic mass of bone and muscle tissue, I began to see the symptoms and progression of MSD as the result of the SLE and MO in six smaller, interactive, interdependent musculoskeletal systems, or "subsystems." Using this diagnostic scheme I knew, for example, that the cause of MSD pain in the front of the head lay elsewhere. Thus, I knew immediately where to palpate for asymmetry, which would guide me to the area(s) where I needed to focus my reversal massage.

Accordingly, in the same way that my reorganization of the musculoskeletal system into subsystems has been useful to me diagnostically, it seems only logical to organize my presentation of the identity and location of symptoms of MSD by subsystem as well, especially given the operating principles of "chain-reactional pulling" and "all-muscles-are-connected." Following my discussion of the symptoms of MSD in the pelvic subsystem in this chapter, I will discuss MSD symptoms in the lumbar subsystem, thoracic subsystem, shoulder girdle subsystem, neck subsystem and finally, the head subsystem in the following chapters. Prefacing the discussion of MSD in each subsystem will be an identification of the major skeletal components and major function(s) of each subsystem.

In my discussion of the progression of MSD causing an individual's symptoms in all of these subsystems, I assume that no shoe lift has been put on the left side, no reversal massage has been performed on any area of the body, and that the individual's history of ARC is average or above average. I also assume that the individual receives adequate nutrition, hydration, and sleep.

Third, my primary focus in Chapters 9 through 14 is the identification, location, and discussion of the more severe symptoms of MSD as I classify them—the symptoms for which most people are likely either to resort to conventional healthcare for consultation or treatment, or to find bothersome or aesthetically displeasing. However, because they are reliable predictors of the more severe symptoms of MSD, I preface the discussion of the more severe symptoms of MSD with mention of some of the asymmetries and other less severe symptoms of MSD to be found in each of the subsystems.

Finally, since I estimate that the functional short leg is the left leg 85% of the time, any reference to the left side should be understood as referring to the functional short leg. Likewise, all references to the right side should be understood as referring to the normal leg.

I believe the pelvic subsystem is the most crucial because first, it occupies a mechanically pivotal area of the body, midway between the head and feet; and second, I believe that within its musculoskeletal mass resides the root cause of the functional short leg and, therefore, of the SLE.

The pelvic subsystem consists of the arrowhead-shaped sacrum, attached to the sides of which are the hip bones (illia), the tailbone (coccyx), two upper leg bones (femurs), each of which is attached to a hip bone, and the bones of the lower legs, ankles, and feet. Last but not least, let's not forget the all the muscles, ligaments, and tendons.

The function of the pelvic subsystem is two-fold. First, the pelvic cavity contains a number of organs critical to reproduction, digestion, metabolism, and other functions. Second, the weight of the entire upper half of the body rests upon the sacrum, an important skeletal intersection between the spine and the pelvis that helps to maintain balance as well as serves as an anchor for activities in the hips, legs and feet.

Mild Symptoms of MSD

The non-painful varieties of asymmetry (stiffness, loss of range of motion or use, differences in size or shape, temperature, and topography) are usually widespread but are especially prevalent in the front of the pelvic region, on the outsides of the thighs, in the buttocks, just below the hips, above the knee caps, in the calves, the tops of the thighs, and in the lower legs. Non-chronic pain (with or without use), numbness, tingling, or burning sensations frequently appear in the buttocks, hamstrings, upper outside thigh, inguinal and groin areas, in the knees (right, left, center, and back), Achilles' tendon, outside of heel, foot (bottom, top, and sides). Painful-with-pressure areas: Inside thighs between knee and groin, outside thighs near the hips, center of buttocks, hip joint, lower pelvic region, inside lower leg, and just below the knee.

Severe Symptoms of MSD

• SACROILLIAC PAIN: The most common symptom of MSD in the pelvic subsystem is in an area commonly referred to as the lower back. The pain in this area is muscle pain resulting from the uneven pull of the contracted muscles involved in the right sacroiliac ("S/I") joint, where the sacrum is connected to the right hip bone. This area is weak from uneven pulling that began in childhood, even before MO, because of the SLE. Not surprisingly, even moderate MO can produce particularly bothersome muscle pain at this joint. S/I pain can even show up in adolescence. When severe S/I pain appears in adults on a chronic basis, it often becomes worse and, in so doing, acquires the name given to the next symptom of MSD: sciatica.

• SCIATICA: In my experience, the "condition" that conventional healthcare professionals call "sciatica" is really "Sacro-Illiac Joint Pain Gone Wild." The unbearable muscle pain associated with that word initially extends from the S/I joint through the buttock and down the outside and front of the leg—usually down the right leg only, in the case of a short left leg, but it can appear in both legs. Later, it can and often does extend clear down to the foot, making the simple act of walking unbearably painful. Conventional healthcare suggests that compression of the sciatic nerve is to blame. I respectfully disagree.

On the basis of my experience with sciatica in my office, I see it as a frequent and predictable extension of S/I pain, whereby the SLE, amplified by MO, takes advantage of the interconnectivity of the muscles down the leg to create one of the most advanced and painful symptoms of MSD in the body. Over the decades, I have successfully treated with a left lift and reversal massage many a patient who was previously given a diagnosis of "sciatica" by conventional healthcare.

The way I envision the process at work here is that the SLE, amplified by MO, causes the muscles of the buttock and the upper muscles of the right leg begin to contract, thereby initiating downward chain-reactional pulling, via the all-muscles-are-connected operating principle. I'll never forget one woman who came into my office in tears, with her leg in so much pain she couldn't use it to propel herself forward and was obliged to walk on her toes. She, too, had been previously diagnosed by conventional healthcare with sciatica. After I fitted her with a left shoe lift and administered a few sessions of reversal massage, she was pain-free and was able to walk and otherwise use her right leg normally. I strongly believe that I have never encountered a true case of "sciatica" in my practice, as conventional healthcare defines it. But, even if I'm wrong, my diagnostic and treatment approaches get rid of the problem just the same.

• HIP PROBLEMS: The uneven muscle tension between the left and right sides of the pelvis, created by the SLE and aggravated by MO, can and often does cause hip pain and, eventually, hip dislocation. Activity involving twisting of the hips in particular can accelerate the advance of MSD. Light palpation of the muscle area on the side of the thigh will usually reveal considerable asymmetry in the form of heat and irregular surface of the muscle tissue. More intense palpation of the muscle tissue close to the hip joint will usually generate pain. As the muscles on the side of the thigh in particular become tauter and exert more and more pull on the hip joint, pain even without palpation is likely. Have you ever noticed times when you can't easily cross your legs when seated, if at all? Regardless of the size of your thighs, if you're unaffected by MSD in the hips, you should be able to put one leg over the other easily. If you can't, you undoubtedly will feel stiffness and pulling along the side of your thighs extending into the buttocks.

Eventually, further contraction of these extremely taut muscles can begin to pull the femur head from its socket (the acetabulum) in the ilium (hip bone). This is the beginning of subluxation and, eventually, possible dislocation in the hip joint. In older people, hip fractures are common, and can occur during an activity as normal as stepping or mis-stepping onto or off a curb or stair step. Though brittle bones due to osteoporosis are often blamed, I believe that a major contributing factor may be the fact that the left hip joint in particular is under tremendous tension from decades of the impact from the SLE and MO, and is therefore predisposed to fracture. As I see it, what also frequently happens is that, as muscle contraction and pulling from the SLE and MO increase in the hip joint, the femur head begins to subluxate and eventually erode, as does the rim of the acetabulum, the socket into which the femur head is normally positioned, and within which the femur head normally rotates as the legs move and twist. As the erosion of the cartilage in this joint begins to become painful, conventional healthcare will issue a diagnosis of osteoarthritis, and hip surgery may loom on the horizon for many.

Because I was able to understand what causes this "osteoarthritis" in the hip, I have been able to initiate reversal through massage and a shoe lift and eliminate the problem. Let me give you one particularly memorable example. A former patient—a housewife—had come to me crying, saying that the doctors wanted to put her in a wheelchair. I calmed her down and asked her to explain. She told me that her X-rays showed that her hip joint was eroding, and that the doctors told her she must be off her feet to heal the joint. I asked her to get her X-rays and bring them to me so I could study the extent of the hip joint erosion in order to know if I could help her. Two days later she returned with her X-rays. The X-rays showed erosion of the femur head and acetabulum cavity rim, commonly diagnosed as osteoarthritis of the hip. Conceptually, I saw the degeneration process in her hip the same as that leading to rupture of a vertebral disc or joint, so I told her that I believed that I could help her.

I studied her previous case history and performed my usual comparative visual and palpation exam, as well as muscle testing. I replaced the old, worn lift on her functional short leg with a new one, and instructed her to refrain from being too active for a month, in order to accelerate the healing process. I then initiated reversal of this common symptom of MSD with my specialized massage.

After two months, she was very grateful to be free of pain. I permitted her short, gentle walks. I palpated her hip joint and found only mild heat and tenderness to the touch. Within another two months, I released her.

• PAINFUL INTERCOURSE: Muscle tension created by the SLE and MO can also affect the area known as the simpus pubis, where the two ischia (butt bones) come together, making sex painful for women in particular.

• DIFFICULT DELIVERY: The SLE and MO in the pelvic area in general can contribute to difficulties in labor and delivery of a baby.

• HEMMORHOIDS: The SLE and MO can affect the musculature in the rectal area, causing protrusion of internal hemorrhoids outside the rectum or, even when there are no hemorrhoids to be found, burning and itching in the rectum.

• SAGGING BUTTOCKS: Have you ever looked in the mirror and lamented the fact that, like several other areas of your body, your buttocks are "going south?" We are told that this change in physique is an evitable part of aging, and, unless we want to buy restrictive undergarments or undergo surgery, we just have to live with it.

Well, I had several patients who didn't want to live with it, but didn't want special clothing or surgery, either. They wanted me to fix the problem, so I did. Let me explain. As with several other areas of the body, the buttocks sag as we get older, but not, in my view, because we get older. What I found in my practice is that the sagging can be reversed by the same type of massage that I used on the rest of my patients. This massage works because the cause of sagging buttocks is the same cause of every other symptom of MSD, a combination of the SLE and MO. As ARC from the use of the legs in various activities transitions into MO, the muscles in and around the buttocks begin to contract, causing the muscular part of the buttocks to become flatter and smaller. The problem with this contraction is that the skin covering the buttock muscles does not also pull inward, but sags or droops downward. As I mentioned in an earlier chapter, it's not unusual to see asymmetry in the buttocks in the form of a dimple in one buttock, reflecting the MO present in that side of the buttock muscles.

At any rate, when I gave particular attention to this area with my massage techniques, I was able to initiate reversal of the contraction process in the buttock muscles, causing them to regain their former contours.

• SAGGING THIGHS: As the muscles of the upper legs, especially those of the inner thighs, contract from the SLE and MO, they begin to flatten out just like the muscles of the buttocks. Similar to what happens with the buttocks, the skin covering the inner thigh muscles does not shrink to conform to the smaller contour of the muscles, but begins to hang loose or sag. This symptom of MSD, too, is usually chalked up to old age. However, as with the sagging of the buttocks, I have reversed this change in physique many times with my massage techniques, eliminating the sagging and restoring tone.

• "RESTLESS LEGS SYNDROME": If you look up the origin of the word "syndrome," you'll find that it is actually a combination of two Greek words that basically translate as "comes with." It's a fancy word to describe a set of symptoms. . .and symptoms they are—symptoms of MSD, that is. If your legs have ever felt restless in this sense, you have experienced a number of irritating feelings in your calves and elsewhere in your legs and have been unable to get comfortable sitting or while attempting to sleep. Recently a drug has come on the market that's supposed to help with these problems. I don't know what the potential side effects of this drug are, or the mechanism by which it attempts to do its job, but what I do know is that I long ago found out how to rid patients of restless legs without drugs.

I believe that the SLE and MO play a causative role in the collection of various uncomfortable sensations referred to as "restless legs." It could be that, for whatever reason and in response to whatever particular physical activity, the calves and other muscles of the legs affected by MO in particular are unable to fully relax, thus producing the uncomfortable restless sensations. Again, whether I'm right or wrong about the exact cause, the responses of my patients with restless legs proved to me that my treatment approach was right on target: reversal massage on specific areas of the body eliminates these uncomfortable sensations.

• MENSTRUAL CRAMPS: Despite the countless drugs on the market and conventional treatments offered to women to relieve the cramping and bloating of the monthly menstrual cycle, I believe that menstrual cramps are caused by the SLE and MO. What's more, I'm here to tell you that I have gotten rid of this bothersome symptom of MSD for a number of women.

What happens during menstruation is like a rehab project going on in the uterus: "Out with the old lining and in with the new." Now, focusing on the blood flow aspect, recall what I mentioned earlier about lower blood pressure readings on my patients after I'd performed my massage in the office. Here's my theory: The pelvic cavity, as well as the organs and specialized anatomical structures located within it, including the uterus, are located at what I call the "Ground Zero" of the SLE. As such, the uterus and the other contents of the pelvic cavity are especially susceptible to stress from the contraction and pulling from MO and the SLE. Therefore, is it not at least plausible that pressure from muscle contraction in the pelvic area can inhibit the muscular contractions of the uterus needed to shed its lining, and that this resistance could produce pressure in the muscle tissues resulting in cramps? Whether I'm right or wrong, I know one thing. . .when I massaged in and around the pelvic areas of the women I treated for menstrual cramps, their cramps disappeared. Not only that, but in a number of cases, since these women had grown to rely on the cramps to herald the onset of their periods, they were surprised to find that their periods had started without their being aware of it until they discovered they were bleeding.

• BLADDER PROBLEMS: Over the years a number of patients came to me complaining of frequent, sudden urges to urinate, sometimes as often as every half-hour. Over the last year or so, I've seen—and so, probably, have you—a TV commercial for a drug to treat this problem, referred to in the commercial as "overactive bladder."

In my practice, I diagnosed and successfully treated this problem differently, without drugs. Based on what I saw as a cause-and-effect relationship between my treatment and cessation of the symptoms of "overactive bladder," I could not reach any other conclusion but that they were a symptom of MSD. Here's how I visualize the situation: Since the pelvic cavity also contains the bladder, it's certainly not far-fetched to envision a situation in which the bladder, crowded in with the other organs like sardines, reacts to unnatural pressure from this crowding and the build-up of constricting muscle tension in the pelvis caused by the SLE and MO. Again, in the patients I treated for this so-called "overactive bladder," the frequent urges stopped altogether. Clearly, this situation presents another choice between eliminating the symptoms by eliminating the symptoms, and eliminating the symptoms by eliminating the cause.

• CONCEPTION PROBLEMS: Once upon a time in my Shelbyville practice, I encountered a couple who had for some time tried to conceive, but repeatedly failed. Their family doctor had ruled out medical problems for both the man and the woman. In examining the woman, I found a tremendous amount of muscle tension in the lower pelvic area, so I performed my massage in the appropriate areas. Perhaps a month or so after I finished treating her, they informed me that she was pregnant. So firmly did she believe that my treatments were responsible that, as she put it, she told her friends that "Dr. Ramsey got me pregnant!"

So, what's my theory on this one? All I can tell you is that, when I examined the patient and found the muscle tension in the pelvis, I was able to visualize how it might be possible for this contracted muscle mass to apply pressure to or squeeze the fallopian tubes and/or the uterus, preventing the unfertilized egg from reaching the area where it could be fertilized by the sperm, or even preventing it from traveling down the fallopian tubes to reach the uterus after having been fertilized. If blood flow could be impeded, it might also be possible that flow through other vessels could be choked off as well. In any event, I reasoned, reversal massage might loosen the tissue enough to allow the fertilization process to continue unimpeded. Was my massage actually responsible? Who knows for sure, but it didn't seem to hurt, and it's certainly something to think about.

• KNEE PROBLEMS: As you'll recall, I went on after my first successful knee joint manipulation to successfully perform many more, learning along the way that what caused the subluxation was the combined action of the SLE and MO, which also created other types of knee problems, also symptoms of MSD. It remains in this section to describe in a bit more detail how the SLE and MO team up to produce a variety of knee problems.

Because of the way the knee joint is designed and constructed, it is particularly vulnerable to the SLE and MO and thus is often victimized by the very muscles which function in its operation. In actuality the knee joint can be looked at as really being composed of three articulating joints, each of which is normally protected from bone-on-bone friction by cartilage. Again, even without the acceleration provided by MO, both knees get off to a bad start because of the initial symptoms of MSD caused by the SLE when we begin to walk as children.

As you'll recall, the left knee is put under unnatural stress from the first effect of the functional short leg, weight imbalance. Over time, uneven muscle tension from physical activity begins to affect the integrity of the joint in another way. Impacted by MO, the space between the bones in the knee joint begins to shorten. As MO progresses, the muscles below the knee team up with the muscles above the knee to pull the bones of the knee out of their normal positions and closer together. Eventually, the ends of the bones, initially covered with protective cartilage, meet and begin to rub and wear on one another. If not checked or reversed, this rubbing will eventually erode the cartilage until none is left, causing the painful bone-against-bone friction and erosion that will, in all likelihood, result in knee replacement.

The right knee joint integrity is threatened on two fronts simultaneously. One is, again, the threat to cartilage from MO. The other threat is to the ligaments and tendons. Given the constant abnormal muscle tension in the right knee from attempting to correct the weight imbalance, MO begins to weaken the muscles of the knee, making them taut and leading to further instability of what is already the most unstable joint in the body. Eventually, this knee will begin to slip out of place, or subluxate. If the uneven pulling and developing muscular dysfunctionality of MSD are not checked or reversed, the patient will begin to experience pain and/ or burning sensations, with or without activity, stiffness, swelling, inflammation, or limited range of motion. Eventually, this knee—as well as the left knee, depending on the nature of activities—can suffer subluxation, dislocation, or a variety of other problems, including osteoarthritis and tears of one or more of the ligaments or tendons. After I furnished them with a lift and reversed the MSD through massage, my patients no longer had knee problems and, as far as I know, avoided surgery.

• CHARLIE HORSES: Leg cramps, especially in the calf muscles, are in my experience yet another symptom of MSD, resulting, again, from the SLE and MO. Over the years, with reversal massage, I have been able to eliminate the tendency to have these sudden and painful cramps, especially in patients who had them frequently.

- ANKLE PROBLEMS: The uneven muscle pull of the SLE and MO make the left ankle more prone to sprain. As I previously mentioned, the pain and discomfort from this type of injury often migrates to areas of the leg above the ankle by chain-reactional pulling. My son experienced a number of left ankle sprains over the years in the course of participating in racquetball, softball, and running. In those cases in which I was available for him and other patients, especially soon after the injury occurred, I was able, with reversal massage, to speed up healing, which normally takes several weeks. Also, over the course of treating a number of ankle sprains, I developed a non-constrictive alternative method of taping the ankle which allows the patient to walk with support, and relatively pain-free.

- FOOT PROBLEMS: As I previously mentioned, as MO begins to amplify the SLE in the pelvic subsystem, the chain-reactional pulling by the dysfunctional muscles begins to extend downward, causing along the way the symptoms of MSD in the hips, thighs, pelvis, knees, calves, and ankles, until it eventually reaches the foot. Since this chain-reactional pulling cannot be transferred from the foot elsewhere, the foot in general and the toes in particular can experience one or all of a number of the symptoms of MSD, including the pain and inflammation that conventional healthcare will call osteoarthritis of the foot. I've already briefly mentioned one of three common symptoms of MSD in the foot, heel pain. Heel pain can also be from a heel spur, a problem I did not happen to treat during my years of practice. However, since reversal massage and manipulation of the heel bone always eliminated the heel pain experienced by my patients, I had no reason to believe that the heel pain they experienced was anything other than a symptom of MSD, resulting from the SLE and MO.

Another is what conventional healthcare calls "plantar fascitis," a painful, burning sensation on the bottom of the arch. This problem, like heel pain, is another symptom of MSD and is the result of the chain-reactional pulling of the dysfunctional muscles that starts in the pelvis due to the SLE and MO.

Generalized pain can occur on top of the foot between the toes and ankle, and along the side of the foot, above the arch. There are other symptoms that can and often do occur, such as a sensation in the back and sides of the heel resembling multiple simultaneous needle pricks. This sensation may come and go, and probably represents inflammation or irritation of the Achilles' tendon by the pulling of taut muscles on the backside of the lower leg, probably involving or irritated by the calf muscle affected by the SLE and MO through chain-reactional pulling. Persistence and intensification of this particular sensation may be a warning that the stage is set for a full-blown rupture or tear of this crucial tendon.

Symptoms of MSD in the toes can take three different forms. First, there can be numbness or pain in one or more of the toes. Second is the barely noticeable but gradual "clawing" effect which can be exhibited by one or more toes, as the chain-reactional pulling continues over time. Third is cramping in the toes.

Finally, there are a couple of symptoms of MSD that show up in the feet that do not involve muscle or joint pain, but can be painful in their own way. Blisters or calluses may develop on the feet especially after, but not limited to, participation in such activities as walking, jogging, running, racquetball, tennis, squash, basketball, soccer, or other activities involving repeated use and pivoting of the legs and feet. Most people are tempted to blame the blisters and calluses on such external factors as poorly fitting shoes or the wrong kind of socks. In my practice, I found that, in reality, many, if not most, of these blisters and calluses are caused by abnormal pressure and inordinate friction due to the SLE. Recall that, as the body attempts to regain balance lost to the SLE, the right leg is unstable, and the right foot is turned outward during walking and other activities using the legs and feet. Depending on what portion of the leg and foot the SLE affects on a particular individual, one or both feet will not hit the ground evenly, making it probable that one area of a foot, whether it be the heel or one or more of the toes, will be exposed to friction where it would it not normally be. Let me give you one example of the SLE in action in this regard.

One woman I treated for neck and shoulder problems had complained that she loved to run but was unable to do so on a regular basis because she always ended up with a blister in the same place on her right foot. After performing reversal massage on the appropriate areas of her legs and fitting her with a left shoe lift, I told her to try running again and let me know what happened. I was not surprised when she told me that when she ran with the lift in her left running shoe, her foot no longer blistered.

Snow skiers might be interested in one phenomenon in their sport that I believe to be a symptom of MSD caused by the SLE in particular. Skiers constantly have to fight to keep their skis parallel, so that they both head in the same direction. Considering the fact that a skier, like most people, wears no shoe lift for the short leg side, and the right (normal) leg tends to be turned outward when standing, it's easy for me to envision the right leg ski also turning outward—to the right—regardless of how the ski boot is constructed. Therefore, I would not be surprised if it skiers could more easily keep their skis parallel by having the correct lift in the short leg ski boot. For that matter, the same principle could apply to other sports requiring the participant to wear specialized footwear, such as ice skating, rollerblading, roller skating, and, perhaps, even water skiing.

In addition to the symptoms of MSD at the aforementioned specific locations between the pelvis and the ends of the toes, one can experience the generalized tactile asymmetry represented as knotty or lumpy areas in the muscle tissue, muscle spasms or cramps that may come and go, or short-lived pain in any given muscle group. Notwithstanding the lesser severity or shorter duration of these milder symptoms of MSD, they are often a predictor of more serious symptoms of MSD to come, unless the MO is offset by reversal massage and the progression of the SLE is slowed by wearing a lift.

CHAPTER 10
The March of MSD:
The Lumbar Subsystem

The lumbar subsystem consists of five lumbar vertebrae, which are the largest and strongest in the spine, as well as the massive musculature that keeps this portion of the spine in alignment. From my perspective, this subsystem has two primary functions. First, it acts as a foundation for the weight of the thoracic, shoulder girdle, neck and head subsystems. Secondly, it provides flexibility for the operations performed by the pelvic subsystem.

Mild Symptoms of MSD

The non-painful varieties of asymmetry (stiffness, loss of range of motion, temperature, or topography) are usually limited to the areas around and extending a short distance from either side of the spinous process at L-4/L-5 and L-5/S-1. Sharp pain with or without use will occur in the same areas as asymmetry. Pain-with-pressure generally tracks the same areas.

Severe Symptoms of MSD

The severe symptoms of MSD found in this subsystem, though few in number, are among the most devastating in the musculoskeletal system in terms of the disability and diminished enjoyment of life they often create. One of the most common and often persistent symptoms of MSD in this subsystem is lower back pain, which is in reality muscle pain resulting from the uneven muscle pulling caused by the SLE and contraction from MO. This pain is usually experienced in two distinct areas of the lower portion of the back, usually on the right side. One is between the fourth and fifth vertebrae of the lumbar section of the spine, referred to as L-4/L-5. The other is the lumbar-sacral joint, which is where the last vertebra of the lumbar spine, L-5, meets the top of sacrum, S-1. As you can now appreciate, L-4/L-5 and L-5/S-1 are likely to be among the areas of the body to experience MSD in the form of severe pain, because of their locations close to the pelvic subsystem—the Ground Zero of the SLE. Because it is located at the point where the entire weight of the upper body rests on the sacrum, L-5/S-1 is very unstable and therefore is particularly vulnerable to stress from uneven pulling by contracted muscles on the right caused by the SLE and MO.

Unfortunately for many, frequent or intermittent pain at L-4/L-5 and/or L-5/S-1 is only the beginning. As MO continues over time and the muscles in this area tighten further, the vertebrae in these locations are prone to subluxate and eventually pinch the nerves coming from the spinal cord. If this subluxation continues, disc problems can result, eventually putting the spinal cord in jeopardy and making the patient a candidate for back surgery.

One event that often pushes a patient who is a borderline candidate for surgery over the edge is lumbar whiplash. Already beset by intermittent pain at L-4/L-5 or L-5/S/1 due to the SLE and MO, a patient in an auto accident suffers aggravation of the pain and deteriorating disc situation from the tremendously stronger and longer-lasting chain-reaction pulling generated by whiplash. Unless this pulling is eliminated by reversal massage and a left lift, the damage to the disc will continue to the point where the patient will have no other conventional healthcare alternative but surgery, sometimes involving fusion of two or more vertebrae. The irony here is that, while fusion surgery may save the spinal cord, it does not stop the gradual pulling of the SLE and MO that necessitated the surgery in the first place, and the patient can experience post-surgery back pain. What's more, fusion usually generates a permanent, and at least partial, disability. In my practice not only did I eliminate the need for surgery and prevent permanent disability by treating the cause of lumbar pain at both of these sites with a lift and reversal massage, I was even able to eliminate post-surgery pain and prevent further surgery and disability the same way. Let me give you one of the more memorable examples from my practice.

I had purchased a small statue of a medieval woman and wanted to have a duplicate made. I didn't know who to call in Shelbyville, so I asked a few people to pass the word around town, hoping that someone who could do the job would contact me. Eventually a local man called me, so I invited him to meet me the next evening at my office. When he arrived, I was sitting on the patio out back. I introduced myself and asked him to sit down. He declined, saying he couldn't sit since his surgery (at L-4/L-5) two years previously for a ruptured disc. He explained that he had been a drywall finisher, which is very strenuous work. I was not surprised that he'd had surgery. At first, he'd been on Workmen's Compensation, until it ran out. Then he was on disability, until it, too, ended. When I met him, he was on welfare.

I suspected I could help him, so we agreed to barter. I would exchange my professional services for his duplication of my statue. The very next day, I evaluated his situation with my usual comparative visual and palpation exams and muscle testing. Then I began reversal massage sessions.

Three months later, he was able to sit, walk, perform yard work, and drive his car. Eventually he was enjoying a normal, active life. Though, I guess, I should not have been surprised, I was nonetheless awed to witness another example of how my massage, supplemented with a lift, had initiated reversal of degenerative damage resulting from years of the SLE and MO, even in a post-surgery situation.

I advised him to ask his orthopedic surgeon if he could return to work, and he came back two days later with the news that his orthopedic surgeon had said he could. And return to work he did, with my invitation to come back to me for treatment if he should begin hurting again. He came back about a year later, complaining of back pain. I treated him as before for a short time, again initiating reversal of the MSD resulting from his return to work as dry wall installer. He went back to work, and I never heard from him again. This patient's situation illustrates the cycle in which contractions are used up by ARC and replaced by my reversal massage. My original massage sessions had initiated reversal, leading to the restoration of his functionality, by essentially putting more contractions on his contraction counter. His return to work as a dry wall installer again used up his available contractions, and, as before, he began to experience pain. When he came back to me, I again put more available contractions on his counter with reversal massage. Though my success with him made him one of my more memorable patients, he was but one of many patients I helped to avoid undergoing initial or continued surgery.

A less common area of back pain and potential disc problems in the lumbar subsystem is at the joint where the first lumbar vertebra, L-1, meets the lowest Thoracic vertebra, T-12. L-1/T-12, like L-5/S-1, is a boundary line (between the lumbar and thoracic subsystems) and is therefore naturally subjected to more stress from the weight of the thoracic subsystem, which contains the internal organs, as well as the shoulder girdle, neck, and head subsystems. The twisting and turning of the shoulder girdle system during use of the hands, arms, and shoulders puts additional stress on this joint. Reversal massage in this area and a left lift made it easy for me to get rid of my patients' muscle pain, thereby enabling them to avoid surgery.

CHAPTER 11
The March of MSD:
The Thoracic Subsystem

The thoracic subsystem is the area of the body commonly referred to as the chest, including the front, back, and sides. The skeletal components are the 12 vertebrae which comprise the thoracic portion of the spine, T-1 through T-12. These vertebrae are the second largest and second strongest in the spine. Next is the rib cage (thoracic cage), composed of 24 ribs. Then there is the sternum, which connects the first six ribs in the center of the upper front chest. Finally, there are various components of the muscular system in this subsystem, including nine different muscles in the thoracic cage alone.

From my perspective, the thoracic subsystem serves two functions. First, it contains and protects a number of internal organs and anatomical features, including the heart, lungs, kidneys, liver, gall bladder, pancreas, spleen and stomach, trachea, esophagus, bronchial tubes, diaphragm, and parts of the colon, or large intestine. Second, it supports the weight of and anchors the shoulder girdle, neck, and head subsystems.

Mild Symptoms of MSD

The non-painful varieties of asymmetry (stiffness, loss of range of motion or use, differences in size or shape, temperature, topography) are found around and adjacent to the rib cage (both sides, front and back), in and around the sternum, between the shoulder blades and the spine, across the top of the chest, just below the arm pits, and along the inside margins of the scapulas. Non-chronic pain (with or without use) is found at the top of the chest, in between both scapulas and the spine, on and below the sternum, and in the rib cage. Pain-with-pressure areas usually track with the non-chronic pain areas, such as around and adjacent to the rib cage (both sides, front and back), in and around the sternum, between the shoulder blades and the spine, across the top of the chest, just below the arm pits, and along the inside margins of the scapulas.

Severe Symptoms of MSD

Because of their size and the massive musculature supporting and stabilizing them, the thoracic vertebrae rarely subluxate—with one exception. That exception is the joint at T-12/L-1 discussed in the last chapter. However, for what the thoracic subsystem lacks in subluxation potential, it more than makes up for it in hosting severe symptoms of MSD.

In Chapter 9, I cited the specific examples of the bladder, the uterus, and the reproductive process in introducing my assertion that contraction or constriction of the body cavity from the SLE and MO can and often does interfere with the normal functioning of organs and crucial bodily processes within that cavity. In this chapter, I again ask you to think outside the organ. It's my assertion, based on my years of practice, that the SLE and MO similarly interfere with the normal functioning of organs, systems, and other bodily processes at work in the thoracic cavity as well. What's different about the Thoracic Subsystem is that the stakes are much higher. Instead of frequent urination, menstrual cramps, and problems conceiving, at risk are such functions as breathing and circulation. Before discussing the organs, systems and other bodily processes affected by MO and the SLE, I want to point out the ways in which the SLE, and the MO in particular, affect the front, sides, and back of the chest.

First, let's remember the structural imbalance resulting from the weight shift to the left initially caused by the SLE after a child takes its first steps. Visualize the organs in the thoracic or chest cavity shifting with gravity, even if ever so slightly, down and to the left. This means that some organs to the top and right may now begin to put pressure on some of the organs to the bottom and left. It's as though you were a passenger standing on the left front side of an elevator filled to capacity. It's crowded, but if no one is touching you, it's bearable for a while. Now, imagine that the elevator tilts slightly to the left and downward. Gravity is forcing the passengers to your right and rear up against you with some pressure. How long could you bear this situation before you begin to malfunction from the stress created by having the weight of those passengers against your body? Eventually, the elevator will be back on track. But the SLE, unless slowed by a shoe lift, will continue to place the organs of the thoracic cavity unnaturally and uncomfortably close to each other. Eventually, something has to give. I'll come back to this later, but, for now, let's put this aspect of the SLE aside, and take a look at the effects of MO, alone, on the thoracic cavity.

The operative rule here is that as the muscles of the arms contract, so does the volume of chest cavity. Let me explain. Over time, as an individual performs numerous types of tasks (again, whether for work, leisure, exercise, or sports) and accumulates repetitive contractions of the muscles of the hands, arms and neck, the nine muscles that support the thoracic cage—particularly those on the front and sides—also are affected, due to the all-muscles-are-connected and chain-reactional pulling operating principles. These chest muscles will then begin to contract and shorten just as the muscles of the arms and legs did. This contraction causes asymmetry and other more severe symptoms of MSD not only in the thoracic subsystem, but also in the shoulder girdle, neck, and head subsystems. It is to the asymmetry and severe symptoms of MSD in the thoracic subsystem created by this contraction that I now turn.

• RECEDING CHEST: One of the most significant—if initially transparent and painless—symptoms of the contraction or shortening of these muscles is a decrease in the volume of the chest cavity. What happens is that the contraction of the muscles on the front and sides of the chest begin to squeeze the chest, especially in the front. Can you imagine wearing a corset, or having a boa constrictor wrapped around your chest? Well, a more gradual, less noticeable version of that squeezing is what you experience over time as the muscles in the front and sides of the chest begin to contract and pull more and more from repetitious activity of the hands and arms. Also, because of the uneven pulling that is characteristic of the SLE, one side—often the right—is squeezed more than the other, creating additional visual and often other types of asymmetry in the front, back, and sides of the chest. In some cases, I have seen this situation aggravated by the effects of congenital malformations of the thoracic cage, such as inward bone development, undersized cage development, an inverted sternum, and even by disease and malnutrition.

To demonstrate how significant receding of the chest can occur unnoticed over time, let me give you one anecdote about a man I know well and have treated for many years. When this man was in his twenties, he had a 44-inch chest, partially due to lifting weights. By the time he was in his forties, even though his weight had not changed appreciably, he inexplicably had dropped two coat sizes, to a size 40. When treating him around that time for symptoms of MSD in the neck and head, I noticed that his chest had receded and he was developing rounded shoulders. Though my massage had already helped some, it was going to take time to accomplish what he needed, so I decided to modify his gravity inversion equipment in order to see what could be accomplished by stretching on this device in a certain way. Not long after a session or two of this stretching, he happened to get fitted for a new suit. To his surprise and mine, he reported that he once more needed a size 44 coat again without any weight gain. When I next saw him, his chest was nowhere near as receded as before, and his tendency toward rounded shoulders had reversed. His neck problems had greatly improved, too. While the degree of reversal through stretching alone on the inversion device overnight was unusual, the symptoms of MSD reflected in his chest were not, exemplifying what the SLE and MO can do to your chest over time.

• CHEST TIGHTNESS: The constriction of the chest cavity can create a feeling of tightness in the center of the chest, especially in or around the sternum. This particular tightness can mimic the pressure or tightness of the chest sometimes experienced during a heart attack. Other areas that often feel tight are located on one or both sides of the rib cage, on the lower edge of and front side of the armpits, and at the lower end of the rib cage on the backside. You may also feel as though a heavy weight is resting across your shoulders.

• CHEST PAIN: As the SLE and MO cause further constriction of the chest, thereby further decreasing the chest cavity volume, an individual will begin to experience advanced symptoms of MSD in the form of pain in most or all of the areas in which chest tightness can be experienced. In addition, pain can be felt in the front, on the edge of the rib cage, across the chest, and clear to one or both shoulders in the area between the breasts and the collar bones. This last area of pain, especially when accompanied by pain in the sternum, can lead some individuals to believe they are experiencing a heart attack. I have seen a number of women who experienced pain in these two areas and, having had a doctor rule out heart problems, were told that the pain was either "in your head" or "anxiety." Also, in at least one case I can recall, a woman had this pain checked out by a doctor who ruled out heart problems. However, she later had trouble getting health insurance because her medical records still reflected pre-existing "heart" problems.

• BREATHING PROBLEMS: The constriction and decreasing volume of the chest cavity can and often does cause shallow, sometimes painful, breathing as the lungs are prevented from fully inflating. Women are particularly prone to experience this symptom. Some may even experience pain in the side of the rib cage when taking a breath. In that case, what may be misdiagnosed as pleurisy is really nothing more than pain in the musculature of the ribs due to the contraction. These symptoms of MSD develop so gradually that you don't initially notice the fact that as time goes on your breathing is increasingly shallow. So obvious is asymmetry in the chest created by this constriction that I can look at a woman's chest from several feet away and tell that she has problems breathing. I often would ask these women if they were having problems breathing. With a look of surprise their faces, they would answer, "Yes. How do you know that?"

Besides limiting how fully you can inflate your lungs, and therefore the amount of oxygen you can take in, the constricted chest cavity causes another problem related to breathing. Think back to an illness you had, perhaps the flu, where you experienced chest congestion and had a great deal of trouble getting rid of that last little bit of mucus, especially from the bronchial tubes. You may even have resorted to over-the-counter or prescription medications to deal with this residual mucus and the frequent, persistent coughing it produced. More likely than not, your inability to cough out this residual mucus was due to the fact that your lungs were unable to fill with enough air to force out the mucus due to the constriction of and decrease in the volume of your chest cavity. In my practice, I took care of this problem with what I call a "percussive" technique that I developed and performed on the upper chest of my patients after massage to initiate reversal of the constriction. These patients were then able to expel the remaining mucus and stop coughing.

• RIB FRACTURES: Have you ever had a sudden onset of excruciating pain in your rib cage only to find, to your puzzlement, that you have a cracked or fractured rib—but no recollection of any trauma that could have caused it? As MO from activities involving use of the hands and arms worsens the contraction and constriction in the rib cage over time, a rib can actually start to bend slightly from the pulling, predisposing the rib to break or crack from a sudden muscular movement. I know of at least one case in which this happened. A man leaped up to slap a volleyball over the net and immediately began to experience the pain from what was later confirmed to be a cracked rib. I have also seen asymmetry in the back side of the rib cage, in the form of one side of the rib cage displaying a bowed or bent configuration in contrast to the normal, more gradually curved contour of the other side of the rib cage.

Again, as with many of the more advanced symptoms of MSD in general, since the symptoms of MSD in the thoracic subsystem take time to develop they frequently go unnoticed. Fortunately these symptoms, as with the other symptoms of MSD, can be eliminated with the use of a left lift and reversal massage.

CHAPTER 12

The March of MSD:
The Shoulder Girdle Subsystem

For the purpose of our discussion, the shoulder girdle subsystem is composed of the shoulder blades, collarbone, a portion of the sternum, the shoulders, arms, hands and, as always, the involved musculature.

One function of the shoulder girdle subsystem is the support of the neck and head subsystems. The other function, which is ironically self-destructing, is to provide, primarily through the two upper extremities, the frequent, enduring, and often intense muscle contractions necessary to lift, pull, swing, push, hold, squeeze, and twist. Consequently, the component extremities, joints, and musculature of this subsystem typically suffer severe symptoms of MSD. What's more, as we will see in the next two chapters, the appearance of symptoms of MSD caused by the MO resulting from the performance of these tasks is not limited to this subsystem.

Mild Symptoms of MSD

The non-painful varieties of asymmetry (stiffness, loss of range of motion or use, differences in size or shape, temperature, or topography) are found along the entire length of one or both arms, from shoulder to wrist, between the shoulder joints and the base of the neck, between the inner margins of the shoulder blades and the spine (left and right), in the shoulder joints, elbow, finger, and thumb joints, tops of forearms, and the insides and outsides of the upper arms. Non-chronic pain (with or without use), numbness, tingling or burning sensations can be found in the tops of the forearms, outsides of the upper forearms, upper arms, shoulders, outer elbows, between the inner margins of the scapulas and the transverse processes, on the tops of the shoulders, in the shoulder joints, between the base of the neck and the shoulder joints, at the wrist, and in the finger and thumb joints. Pain-with-pressure can be found around the elbow, in the upper and lower forearms, insides and outsides of the upper arms, tops of the shoulders, in the shoulder joint, between the inner margins of the scapulas and the spine, and in the finger and thumb joints.

Severe Symptoms of MSD

Because the progression of the severe symptoms of MSD within the shoulder girdle subsystem is from the top downward, I will discuss the symptoms in that order. As always, recall that the aforementioned asymmetry and other less severe symptoms of MSD will usually precede the severe symptoms of MSD that follow.

• SHOULDER PAIN: As the MSD continues its progressive march, the muscles on the backside, between the shoulder blades (scapulas) will begin to hurt during use or even when not in use.

MO will create muscle pain in the areas around and just below the shoulder joint. Also, even before the onset of this shoulder pain, it is not uncommon for the muscles involved in the shoulder joint to have begun the subluxation process. As the humerus, or upper arm bone, is gradually pulled out of its normal anatomical position in the shoulder joint, there is no pain, but as the erosion of the joint due to subluxation continues, this joint will become painful and will be diagnosed by conventional healthcare as "osteoarthritis" of the shoulder. Over time, I was actually able to confirm, through palpation and visual exams for asymmetry, subluxation of the shoulder joint. After preparing the joint with reversal massage, I was able to manipulate it back into place.

In some cases, as with subluxated vertebrae in the spine, marginal shoulder subluxation may be reversed by inadvertent auto-manipulation.

For example, let's say you attempt to remove the wrinkles in the front of your shirt by placing your thumbs inside the left and right sides of the waistband of your pants and sliding each thumb around to the back. If the muscles in the subluxated shoulder joint are loose enough, you will hear a muffled "pop," signaling a successful, if unintentional, attempt at manipulating the shoulder joint back into place—without your realizing it was subluxated in the first place.

The reverse is not true, however. Just as there is no pain during the subluxation of the shoulder joint, there is no sound effect as any of the other joints subluxate. Also, depending on the particular state of the muscles involved in the shoulder, or any other joint, the success of the manipulation, intentional or not, may be short-lived. If the tension resumes, the joint may silently and painlessly re-subluxate, again, unbeknownst to the patient until the next muffled "pop" heralding another successful albeit inadvertent auto-manipulation. This in-again, out-again cycle can last for years.

Finally, MO can cause muscle pain in the upper chest area close to or around the clavicle joints.

• ROTATOR CUFF PAIN: While usually not sufficient to produce a tear of this muscle, MO from certain tasks or motions of the upper arm directly involving or indirectly affecting the rotator cuff muscle will produce mild-to-moderate, and possibly persistent, pain. I was able to correct this problem with manipulation of the associated shoulder joint.

• "TENNIS ELBOW": So-named because it frequently occurs in the elbow of the racquet hand of avid tennis players, it can also plague players of racquetball, squash, baseball, softball, or even piano. However, since it is a symptom of MSD caused by MO in the affected arm, it can also result from a variety of work, leisure, or other non-sporting activities. Conventional healthcare and I agree in principle that (1) the main symptom is pain when attempting to grip and twist, squeeze or turn (as in turning a doorknob) shaking hands, or using a hand-held stapler; (2) the cause is overuse of the affected arm in one or more of the referenced activities; (3) rest of the arm is an important factor in getting rid of the problem. However, conventional healthcare and I disagree somewhat on the precise cause and the most effective way to rid a patient of tennis elbow.

Conventional healthcare attributes this problem to tendon damage from overuse of the arm. I believe that the main culprit is, as with other problems caused by MO, a contracted muscle or set of muscles pulling on and aggravating the tendon(s), as opposed to actual tendon damage. Also, in my experience, there is a component of muscle dysfunctionality or weakness in addition to, and far overshadowed by, the pain. I say this because, in my practice, I have found that with just a few minutes of reversal massage in certain areas of the arm affected by tennis elbow, grip strength would increase and pain with or without use would drastically decrease. If the tendon were truly damaged, how could it repair itself in just a few minutes? It was clear to me that what really was happening was that the massage reversed the contraction in the muscles, thereby lengthening them and decreasing the pull on the tendon. Predictably, if the patient ignored my instruction to rest the arm and immediately resumed normal use after my initial massage, the pain and decrease in grip strength would return. When I again massaged the area, the pain again would decrease and the grip strength would increase.

• CARPAL TUNNEL SYNDROME: Many in conventional healthcare agree that carpal tunnel syndrome is caused by repetitive stress to the hands, usually in the workplace, or, more recently, from computer use. Everyone in healthcare has a solution, ranging from surgery to sever the trans-carpal ligament thought to be putting pressure on the median nerve in the carpal (wrist) canal, to drugs, to immobilization of the affected area with wrist splints or wraps.

For years I was ridding my patients of the pain, tingling, numbness, and loss of grip strength characterizing this problem before I realized it even had a name! When I discovered it indeed had a name, I began reading about it.

I remember reading a report many years ago by some medical researchers who had tried for about twenty years to prove that median nerve compression even actually occurred. They were unable to do so. Is it that the compression really does exist, and they just couldn't find it, or is median nerve compression a phantom?

I don't know the answer to that question, but, on the basis of my experiences in my practice, I can tell you that I believe that what conventional healthcare calls "CTS" is actually another severe symptom of MSD caused in the same way that other joint problems in the body are caused, by the SLE and MO. My belief is based on the fact that I got rid of CTS with my massage technique applied to one particular place on the arm, supplemented only by resting and/or reducing the usage of the arm.

• OSTEOARTHRITIS IN THE HAND: In addition to the tendency to drop things or the inability to hold onto things for very long that frequently come with MSD in the wrist or carpal tunnel syndrome, a patient may find that one or more of the joints of the thumb or fingers has become painful, and that patient most likely will be diagnosed by conventional medicine with osteoarthritis of the hand. As I explained, earlier, "osteoarthritis" in these and the other joints of the body is actually a symptom of MSD, from either subluxation or erosion of the joint, or both. Not only have a number of my patients been diagnosed by conventional healthcare with the condition of osteoarthritis in the hand, but, occasionally, due to my own MO, I have also experienced pain in one of my thumb joints. Again, knowing where and how to massage and manipulate eliminated this problem for my patients and me—although, I must admit, I had to have someone help me with the manipulation, since it's difficult to self-manipulate the joints of your own hand!

• ROUNDED SHOULDERS: As chain-reactional pulling begins to pull the neck downward and inward, it also begins to pull the shoulders forward and inward. The resulting change in physique is called "round shoulders" due to the fact that an imaginary line drawn between the tops of the shoulders is curved instead of straight. Round shoulders is less a severe symptom of MSD than an indicator of what is happening in the rest of the chest. From my experience, this particular symptom of MSD, as with the others of the thoracic subsystem, is especially common in women. One reason may be the fact that, in addition to work performed outside the home, women who are also mothers perform additional contractions with the muscles of the arms, hands, and shoulders in breastfeeding, picking up and holding children for long periods of time, cleaning, cooking, and laundering. These additional tasks are bound to accelerate the onset of rounded shoulders, as well as accelerate the decrease in the chest cavity volume.

Over the years, I would learn that, as with the other symptoms of MSD, I was able to literally straighten out this rounded shoulder condition as far as a given patient wanted. However, my first opportunity to see just how far I might be able to take it with this symptom of MSD made me wonder. A woman in her seventies was brought to me by her husband. He told me that he wanted to see how much I could straighten her rounded shoulders. At this point in my career, though my previous successes in reversing other changes in physique due to MO encouraged me to give it a try, I really wasn't sure how much I could do for her, given her age. Undaunted, I began a series of reversal massage sessions targeting what I calculated to be the key muscle groups.

After the initial series, both her husband and I were encouraged to see her shoulders receding slightly. At this point, the woman wanted to quit, since, again, coming to me was his idea, not hers. Her husband, however, insisted that she continue the treatment. After a number of subsequent sessions, both her husband and I were amazed with the results. At the point at which her husband was satisfied and discontinued the sessions, my massage had reversed this symptom of MSD to the extent that her shoulders had moved almost all the way back to normal.

Just as I had seen how even young people could suffer from severe symptoms of MSD, my experience with this patient demonstrated that advanced age was not a barrier to elimination of the severe symptoms of MSD, either.

CHAPTER 13
The March of MSD:
The Neck Subsystem

Skeletally, the neck subsystem consists of the seven vertebrae known as C-1 through C-7. Because they are the smallest and weakest vertebrae in the spine, they are particularly prone to slippage or subluxation. As you'll recall, C-1 and C-2, the atlas and axis, are somewhat different from the other vertebrae in form and function. The head rests on the atlas, the bony, ring-shaped platform. The atlas, in turn, sits atop the second vertebra, the axis, the main distinguishing feature of which is the bony knob, around which the head and atlas pivot. This combination of the atlas and axis allows the head to move from side to side as well as up or down. Also included in this subsystem are the muscles and ligaments that function to support and stabilize the head and cervical spine.

The two functions of the neck subsystem are to balance and support the head and to give the head flexibility in movement. Unfortunately, the very design of the atlas and axis combo makes it a high-maintenance structure. Even on the best of days, the supporting muscles of the cervical spine struggle to maintain stability and balance of the head. So when the SLE and MO in the shoulder girdle subsystem travel up into the neck via chain-reactional contraction pulling not only is the performance of this balancing act compromised but the entire subsystem begins to display increasingly severe symptoms of MSD.

Mild Symptoms of MSD

The non-painful varieties of asymmetry (stiffness; loss of range of motion or use; differences in size, shape, temperature, topography) are found along the entire length of the neck as well as in the front and both sides, with mild stiffness and shorter turning radius and differences in length and topography being most common. Non-chronic pain (with or without use) can develop, usually for short periods of time, in most areas of the neck. Painful-with-pressure areas emerge along the sides of the neck and the back of the head.

Severe Symptoms of MSD

• CERVICAL SUBLUXATION: Apart from the fact that the cervical vertebrae are smaller and weaker than their thoracic and lumbar counterparts, the musculature in the neck that is supposed to support and stabilize them is compromised by the SLE and MO exported from the shoulder girdle subsystem. In other words, the neck pays for the overindulgence of the hands, arms, and shoulders.

The main area in which the neck pays is near the top. The triad joint formed by head, C-1, and C-2 is particularly unstable. When subjected to uneven muscle pulling between the left and right sides of the neck generated by the SLE and MO in the shoulder girdle subsystem, not only are C-1 and C-2—the atlas and axis— easily subluxated but the head, prone to slip off center of the atlas, frequently rotates and tilts to one side.

While in my experience subluxation is uncommon below C2, it can and sometimes does occur at C-3/C-4. It is also possible, given the amplification of SLE over time by persistent and severe MO, for several of the cervical vertebrae to be in a subluxated state simultaneously. One memorable example that comes to mind is the case of a service industry worker I briefly treated. For well over a decade, the demands of the job required the performance of repetitive tasks with both hands while taking phone calls, forcing this individual to hold the receiver clamped between head and shoulder. A few hours after my initial reversal massage session the patient made an unconscious turn of the head, setting off an unanticipated but successful auto-manipulation of three or four cervical vertebrae in rapid succession evidenced by muffled, machine-gun-like popping sounds. Another patient I have treated has for years experienced the same rapid, multiple-vertebrae auto-manipulation in both the cervical and thoracic spine when sneezing in a bent-over position.

• CERVICAL DISC PROBLEMS: As MO in the hands, arms, and shoulders increases in severity, subluxation of the cervical vertebrae advances into various problems with the discs at C-3/C-4. As with the lumbar spine, these disc problems can and often do result in surgery to protect the spinal cord.

• STIFF NECK: A neck that feels stiff and often painful can result from the SLE and MO exported from the shoulder girdle subsystem in at least five different ways, each a pathway for chain-reactional muscle pulling to travel up into the neck. One would be the normal tautness attributable to MO that may, because of the SLE, cause more stiffness on one side than the other. A second is through whiplash. A third is lying down or sleeping several hours in a position that constantly pulls on one side of the neck, such as when you lie down and support your neck with your hand or the armrest of a couch. A fourth is by holding a phone in the curve of your neck for any length of time. And a fifth is to talk on any type of phone for a long period of time.

A stiff neck can also affect the circulatory system, particularly the blood flow in the carotid arteries. Some of my patients with an especially stiff and shortened neck reported that when they suddenly turned their head quickly to one side or the other, they briefly felt light-headed, or as if they were about to faint. As I see it, the most likely explanation for this is that the already severe muscular tension in the front and sides of the neck was made worse when turning, effectively impeding or decreasing the blood flow through one or both carotid arteries, the major suppliers of blood to the brain.

• SAGGING SKIN: At the same time you're acquiring a set of rounded shoulders because of the effect MO in the thoracic subsystem has on your chest cavity, other structural changes, manifested as negative developments in your physique, are often occurring in the neck subsystem due to MO exported from the thoracic and shoulder girdle subsystems.

First, you notice that the skin under your chin begins to sag. Second, either the skin in your neck also begins to sag, your neck begins to look fatter, or both. Third, your neck appears to be growing shorter. Fourth, if you look at the side of your neck in a mirror, and then compare what you see to other people's necks—and not necessarily younger people—you'll notice that your neck no longer seems to rise straight up from your shoulders, but appears to be angling forward. If you notice one or more of these changes in your physique and begin searching for answers, don't bother knocking at the door of "old age." Instead you can thank MO in the thoracic and shoulder girdle subsystems for each and every one of these changes. How does this happen?

Two phenomena are occurring simultaneously to generate these changes. First the contour of your skin generally tends to follow that of the muscle tissue that lies underneath it. However, though the musculature of the neck begins to tighten and contract from MO generated by and exported from the shoulder girdle subsystem, the skin overlying that musculature does not shorten, thus giving the sagging effect.

Meanwhile, long-term chain-reactional pulling has shortened the cervical spine, causing the neck to start moving forward and downward into the chest. The overall visual effect is much like that of a turtle retracting its head into its shell. As a result, the bottom of the jaw is now closer to the chest and the top of the shoulders, and the skin surrounding the neck sags. With the neck now pulled forward due to contracted, shortened muscles and a compressed or shortened cervical spine, the area of the neck between the bottom of the jawbone and the top of the shoulders still has the same amount of skin covering it as it did when the muscles were longer and larger, enhancing the sagging appearance.

To the extent these changes eventually become noticeable, they, too, are written off as "old age," or the extra skin is donated to a plastic surgeon. In my experience however, the musculoskeletal reality is that these changes are not badges of old age, but symptoms of MSD, due to the SLE and MO. Look around and you'll see older people whose necks are just as straight and slender as those of younger people and whose chin and neck skin is just as taut as that of younger people. These people are indisputably older, so the sagging neck cannot be purely a result of age. These older people have managed to avoid the SLE and MO that others have not.

There is a "good news, bad news" aspect to these symptoms of MSD. The bad news is that, as we shall see in the head subsystem, these changes are more than just skin deep, as their appearance signals a predisposition to other more severe symptoms of MSD. The good news, as with the other symptoms of MSD I've treated, is that these changes are reversible. For many patients, I removed the sagging skin and shortened, fattened, bent neck, just like the woman whose round shoulders I helped straighten, all by knowing where and how to massage.

• HICCUPS AND MORE: As with the other subsystems, I have had the rare opportunity to encounter and successfully treat, through inspired experimentation, patients suffering from some of the more unusual symptoms of MSD in the neck subsystem. Given the numerous examples of extreme tension in the neck I have observed in many patients over the years, as well as the variety of critical body functions in which the throat muscles play a part, I am not surprised as I look back that, using nothing more than my specialized massage techniques, I have successfully treated and eliminated persistent hiccups, difficulty in swallowing, laryngitis and/or speaking with difficulty, frequent sensitive or sore throats, and persistent, unexplained coughing or feeling the need to clear the throat.

Of these patients, I remember in particular a man who came to me complaining of frequent, persistent hiccups. This man worked in a manufacturing plant, performing tasks requiring repeated use of his hands, arms, and shoulders. From his repeatedly positive

responses to my treatment, it was clear to me that the MO resulting
from his work had traveled up into his neck, stimulating whatever
mechanism is necessary to produce a hiccup. After a session or two
in my office, his hiccups stopped. As he accumulated additional
repetitive contractions from performing his job, his hiccups would
return, and I would again put a stop to them with reversal massage.
My experience with this patient again illustrates the cycle in which
ARC took available contractions off his counter, and I put them
back on with my massage, reducing his hiccup count in the process!

CHAPTER 14
The March of MSD:
The Head Subsystem

Skeletally, the head subsystem consists of the skull, which in turn includes eight cranial bones and 14 facial bones, including the upper and lower jawbones. Contained within the facial bones are the sinus cavities and the boney part of the nose. The non-skeletal components include the eyes; teeth, tongue and other features of the mouth; the pituitary gland; the components of the ear; and all the involved musculature.

From the standpoint of joint activity the skull sits atop the ring-like C-1 vertebra, the atlas, which in turn sits atop the C-2 vertebra, the axis. When functioning normally, this arrangement allows the head to rotate right and left as well as up and down. The other moving joint is the temporomandibular joint, which facilitates the opening and closing of the jaw.

Functionally, this subsystem provides a protective housing for the brain, from which the spinal cord descends through the entire length of the spinal canal of the spinal column, along the way branching out from between the left and right sides of the vertebrae in the form of the spinal nerves, thus providing energy to various parts of the body. The skull cavity also provides partial protection for the nasal passages, eyes, and ears. Thus, the head subsystem houses the organs of the six senses: vision, smell, taste, hearing, touch, and balance, as well as the crucial components of the nervous system that monitor these and other functions in the body.

Mild Symptoms of MSD

The non-painful varieties of asymmetry (stiffness, loss of range of motion or use, differences in size or shape, temperature, and topography) are most commonly found in or around the temporomandibular joint; along the jawline; in the cheek, the eyelids, the forehead; in the sides and the back of the head; above, below and around the ears; above the eyes; and in the teeth. Also, one ear will appear to sit higher on the head, as well as more forward, and the opening of the ear canal will be wider on one ear. Non-chronic pain (with or without use) is usually found in or around the temporomandibular joint, along the jawline, back of the head, in the teeth, gum line, cheek, temples, around the ear. Pain-with-pressure is usually found at the back or base of the head, and the cheek.

Severe Symptoms of MSD

The head subsystem is a showcase for many of the more severe symptoms of MSD for three reasons. First, the head is, for my purposes, a functional extremity just like the hands and feet even if it is not considered so anatomically. As we have seen with the hands and feet, the head, including the musculature, organs, and sensory processes operating within it, is the ultimate victim of the chain-reactional pulling facilitated by the all-muscles-are-connected musculoskeletal operating principle. Second, in contrast to the relatively limited prospects for the SLE and MO to wreak havoc in the hands and feet, there simply are more targets of opportunity in the head with the musculature, organs, and sensory processes in operation there. Third, while we have seen how the neck subsystem is itself a victim of MSD, it is at the same time an exporter of MSD, as the strong musculature of the neck helps amplify and transfer to the head the powerful chain-reactional pulling generated by the shoulder girdle caused by the SLE and MO in the hands arms and shoulders.

In pointing out the various locations at which and ways in which the SLE and the effects of MO literally "come to a head" in this subsystem, I'll start where I left off in the neck subsystem, at the jawline.

• TMJ SYNDROME: If you have ever suffered from this severe symptom of MSD, you have experienced one or more of the following: intermittent or chronic headache pain; pain in the cheek, temple, or ear; difficulty in fully opening—or outright locking of—the jaw; popping or clicking noises when you open your jaw; tinnitus (ringing in the ears) or various types of high pitched "whining" or "fluttering" sounds. No doubt when you consulted a doctor or researched the Internet, you were told or read that these phenomena can be attributed to trauma, excessive chewing (especially gum), osteoarthritis, psychological stress, grinding your teeth, or bite problems. Just as surely, you were told about or found out about a number of treatment alternatives, including surgery, medications, and resting the jaw muscles. As you may have surmised from my very reference to TMJ syndrome as a symptom of MSD, my success in treating patients with this problem has given me a different view of its cause and treatment.

In the cases of TMJ syndrome I have treated, including one in which I associated with a dentist, I found success using nothing more than the same tools I used with other symptoms of MSD: comparative visual and palpation exams, muscle testing, and specialized massage. Though TMJ syndrome was an exciting challenge at first, I realized that I was successful in eliminating it with these tried-and-true tools because TMJ problems are primarily the end result of the SLE and MO reaching up from the neck subsystem from activities in the shoulder girdle subsystem. As muscles in the neck begin to contract and pull as a result of hand, arm, and shoulder MO, the chain-reactional pulling and all-muscles-are-connected principles facilitate the extension of this pulling upward into the muscles around and underneath the ear, eventually affecting the operation of the temporomandibular joint. While this joint is the primary and often initial target, the chain-reactional pulling continues to advance around the jaw line and into the cheek muscles, as well as to the side of and above the ear.

As with the knee and hip, conventional healthcare focuses on the temporomandibular joint in isolation, and does not, as I do, think far outside the joint in searching for causation.

As a result, excessive chewing is put on the list of top suspects. This is curious to me because conventional healthcare takes just the opposite approach in identifying the major contributing factor in the cause of tennis elbow and carpal tunnel syndrome: overuse of the muscles outside the affected joint. I believe that the causative role of either excessive chewing, or chewing, period, in TMJ problems is minimal. First of all, the muscles that allow us to chew are designed to chew, just as the muscle tissue in the heart is designed to beat millions of times during our lives. We have all been told for decades that, for proper digestion of our food, we should chew each bite a certain number of times, like twenty-two. Do you chew each bite of your food twenty-two times? Just the mental task of counting to twenty-two each time you take a bite is enough to give you a headache! And besides, how do you explain TMJ problems in people who almost never chew gum, or the lack of TMJ issues in people who do chew gum or tobacco products? Is it not possible that gum-chewing perhaps does little more than use up the muscle contractions we don't perform by not chewing each bite even remotely close to twenty-two times? While you chew on that, allow me to continue. . .

Stress and trauma certainly can play a role, but not a determinative one, I think. Stress can and does marginally further tighten already taut chest, shoulder, and neck muscles, but I think it's important to consider the condition of those muscles before stress acts on them. Trauma also may have more of an impact on causation, depending on the severity and type; a jab to the jaw or cervical whiplash will, I believe, aggravate a pre-existing taut set of muscles in the chest, shoulder girdle, and neck, possibly causing a temporary outbreak of additional symptoms of TMJ syndrome. Again, it's important to remember that TMJ syndrome, like all other joint and muscular symptoms of MSD, is created over time through repetitive activities.

As for bite problems being a causative factor, I submit that the chicken is being confused with the egg. As I will discuss in the next section, bite problems and clenching of teeth are much more likely co-symptoms of TMJ syndrome, caused by the SLE and MO, than to cause TMJ syndrome by themselves. However, despite the fact that it was always more work and often took longer—because it is a symptom of more advanced MSD—I have successfully gotten rid of TMJ syndrome with my specialized massage techniques.

• DENTAL PROBLEMS: The same chain-reactional pulling process that causes TMJ syndrome can cause other severe symptoms of MSD in the form of bothersome misalignments in the structures of the jaw, teeth, and gums. Musculature involved in the front and sides or margins of the jaw can be intermittently painful or spasm. The pulling can cause teeth to start crowding, sometimes chronically, making it difficult to get even waxed floss in between them. It can also create a temporary feeling of tooth sensitivity for which there is no dental basis. The muscle tissue above the gum line can become so inflamed that even cool food can generate pain of a type usually associated with an exposed root. The muscle tension can be severe enough to cause the gums to bleed spontaneously even where there are no periodontal problems. Finally, given the uneven pulling on and in the jaws, the bite can be affected in at least two ways. First, the alignment of the teeth can be thrown off. Second, this pulling can cause a change in the angle at which the jaws come together, resulting in grinding or erosion and eventually, perhaps, chipping or fracturing of one or more of the back molars. These problems can come and go with the fluctuating severity of TMJS, which in turn fluctuates with increasing and decreasing tension in the jaw area.

• HEARING PROBLEMS: Over the years, many patients on whom I performed my specialized massage techniques specifically to deal with MSD in one or more of the other subsystems got up from my treatment table saying they could hear better. I don't know exactly how my massage techniques have this effect, but I think it has something to do with the fact that the size of the opening of the ear canal is usually larger for one ear than the other, due, in my estimation, to greater muscle tension and pulling on that side.

Hearing specialists may debate with me about this, but I believe the ear with a smaller opening will not let in sound as well. Or perhaps my massage somehow positively affects the inner organs of hearing. Regardless, my former patients' unsolicited positive feedback cannot be ignored.

Tension in the neck traveling up underneath the ear can produce a noticeable partial temporary loss in hearing. When the tension is released through my reversal massage, the ear can once again "pop," similar to the experience of intermittent ear popping when you have a cold or are flying in an airplane.

• SINUS PROBLEMS: As my palpation of the faces of a number of patients has revealed, the chain-reactional pulling that causes the symptoms of MSD often extends to the muscle tissue on either or both sides of the nose, aggravating or facilitating the clogging of the sinuses. In some people, the nasal passages can become so clogged that they are really breathing through only one nasal passage. Frequently I saw that a patient's nostril on one side would be larger than on the other. This suggested to me that the passageway with the smaller opening was clogged and that the larger opening on the other side was the natural result of the body's attempt to compensate for the loss of oxygen intake on the other side. Regardless, with my massage techniques, I have reversed the muscle contraction causing this problem for many patients, allowing them to breathe easier.

• VISION PROBLEMS: As the muscle tension extends up the side of the face adjacent to the outside corner of one or both eyes, the functioning of the muscles controlling the movement of the eyelids and the eye can be affected. On many patients, I have seen one eyelid twitch or spasm, or even droop a bit. Also, especially with contact lens wearers, it appears that the shape of the cornea can be slightly altered by an episode of particularly aggravated muscle tension transferred from the neck, so that for a period of time, focus is not as sharp as usual. I've also seen redness, and had complaints of a "scratchy" feeling with or without redness, in either side of the whites of the eye due to swelling of the small blood vessels there and apparently caused by extraordinary pulling on the adjacent muscles. Here, again, my specialized massage eliminated these problems.

• AGING IN THE FACE: In my experience, as with every other area of the head subsystem, the face displays the symptoms of MSD created by the exportation of chain reaction pulling from the neck and shoulder girdle subsystems. The particular symptom of MSD displayed in the face is asymmetry. The overall effect here is that the patient, especially a woman, can look much older than her true age from sheer muscle tension. Innumerable women who received my reversal massage would look younger in the face by a decade or more.

• SUBLUXATION: Theoretically, any or all of the cervical vertebrae can subluxate and cause disc problems, but I seldom encountered subluxation in the head subsystem outside of the head itself, C-1 and C-2. The instability inherent in the arrangement between these skeletal components makes the head especially prone to chain-reactional pulling, so it was not unusual for me to find a patient's head rotated to the left or right, tilted downward to the left or right, or a little of both. This same pulling force also will often force slippage at the atlas/axis interface. I have been able to restore the head to a front-facing, upright position with massage, usually within few minutes. However, to reseat the atlas on the axis, I would have to perform both massage and manipulation.

• MIGRAINES AND OTHER HEADACHES: Many, if not most, of the patients who came to me for frequent, severe headaches had already been to conventional healthcare. After their expensive and time-consuming diagnostic test results came back negative, these patients were told that their headaches could not be explained. Over the years, I got rid of headaches in various locations and of all degrees of severity, including the mother of all headaches, the dreaded migraine. Before I talk a bit more about migraines and headaches in general, let me describe what I have come to know as the four main causes of headaches. In decreasing order of frequency, they are musculoskeletal, emotional, physiological, and pathological.

By "musculoskeletal" headaches, I of course mean another example of one of the more severe symptoms of MSD. By "emotional" headaches, I mean those caused by the aggravation of pre-existing symptoms of MSD by emotional stress. I'll come back to this shortly. By "physiological" headaches, I mean those which are or can be caused by malfunctioning body processes or systems, such as low blood sugar or hypoglycemia, resulting from improper eating or, more often, missing meals. By "pathological" headaches, I mean those caused by brain tumors or disease. These, of course, I cannot help, and I have referred a few patients to conventional healthcare for consultation. However, in my experience, brain tumors are the least common cause of frequent headaches.

In my practice, I have found that a thorough history is particularly important in diagnosing the cause of and eliminating headaches. This is because in some cases, a person can have two headaches in the same period of time that have two unrelated causes. For example, the headache of a patient who is both a poor eater and a sufferer of MSD can be physiological in origin, musculoskeletal in origin, or both. In that case, in order to cover all bases, both reversal massage and dietary changes may be necessary.

Though I have counseled many patients on nutrition, thereby helping them to understand the origin of and eliminate with self-help their hypoglycemic, or physiological, headaches, it was the headaches in the last two categories, musculoskeletal and emotional headaches, that I most often dealt with and eliminated in my practice.

If you research the word "migraine" you'll find that it roughly translates to "half of the head," referring to the fact that those suffering what they believe to be a migraine headache usually—but not necessarily always—experience pain on either the left or right side of the head. Though conventional healthcare does not claim a cure for migraines, it offers many theoretical explanations for the excruciating, throbbing head pain that increases with activity, the sensitivity to light and sound, "aura" in the form of flashes of light or needle-point sensations in an arm or leg, or nausea that are most often cited as symptoms of a "migraine." Conventional healthcare also offers a variety of drugs said to help reduce the frequency and severity of these symptoms.

As with the so-called carpal tunnel and restless legs syndromes, I was getting rid of my patients' migraine and other musculoskeletal headaches before I knew the word "migraine" existed with the same specialized exam and massage techniques I used to eliminate the other symptoms of MSD I cite in this book.

To me, a musculoskeletal headache is a musculoskeletal headache. The fact that some, like the migraine, have worse pain than others or are accompanied by other unusual symptoms doesn't change my opinion. Based on my experience, the migraine and the other headaches are just additional examples of the severe symptoms of MSD caused by the combined action of the SLE and MO exported from the shoulder girdle and neck subsystems.

I can't tell you with certainty why the sensitivity to light and sound, the "aura," or the nausea often accompany a migraine, but I don't really need to know why, either. What I do know is that, given my success with eliminating the other more severe symptoms of MSD in the head and elsewhere with the same approach— massage—I'm not surprised by the appearance of these phenomena.

First, let's remember where migraines are experienced: in the head, a functional extremity, and the last, most unfortunate victim of severe chain-reactional muscle pulling that originates in the shoulder girdle subsystem, sent upward by the neck subsystem, and caused by ARC of the muscles of the hands, arms, and shoulders.

Second, though I have not emphasized it until now, the muscle pull on the back and sides of the head appears, from my experience in palpating the heads of many patients, to cause considerable asymmetry, inflammation, and pressure on the sides, back, and top of the skull bones by pulling on the muscles attached to the skull. Given the fact that the brain and organs of sight are located inside the skull, and my observations that the chain-reactional pulling has caused a number of my patients to experience pain in the forehead and/or eye sockets sufficient to make them feel that their eyeballs were going to pop out of their heads, is it all that farfetched to suspect a possible connection between the muscle tension and pressure on the skull and the sensation of seeing flashing lights? Also, if your eyeballs feel that way, it's not surprising that you'd be hypersensitive to light and seek out a dark room.

Also, given the fact that, as I've already related, patients with milder contraction pulling had their hearing improved after my massage, is it not conceivable that the extraordinary tension on the side of the head can impact the hearing process in a way which makes it hypersensitive to noise?

So what could explain the nausea? Well, as you can read for yourself, it is a known potential reaction to pain. And what of the needle-point sensations in an arm or leg? These may be either different expressions of MSD-based pain, or perhaps the result of pressure on the brain.

Whether I'm right or wrong in my theories about the reasons for phenomena that often accompany a migraine doesn't change the fact that my massage techniques not only eliminated migraines in many patients, but also decreased the frequency and severity of the migraines when they did return. Let me furnish but one memorable example among many.

Recall my patient who experienced a successful, spontaneous auto-manipulation of several cervical vertebrae after only the first or second visit. Something else happened after that patient's two visits. That patient's migraines didn't return for a significant period of time, and when they did, they weren't nearly as severe even though I understood that the physical and other stresses this patient was enduring before visiting me continued or worsened after the second visit. The reduction in frequency and severity of migraines in this person was, in my view, neither coincidental nor exceptional—even after only two visits. Circumstances didn't allow me to follow up with this patient for very long after the two sessions but, had I the opportunity to continue with the reversal massage, I know from the histories of my other migraine patients that I could have further reduced the frequency and severity of this patient's migraines.

Non-migraine musculoskeletal headaches are also caused by the SLE and MO exported from the shoulder girdle subsystem, and can appear at various places in the head, such as the forehead, back of the head, or in the temple(s). These, too, are effectively eliminated by my reversal massage.

Emotional headaches are, in my view, the result of aggravation of normally asymptomatic MSD in the form of usually painless chain-reactional pulling that extends up into various places on the head. As I like to say, "The mind speaks to the body." Emotional and/or psychological stress causes already taut muscles in the shoulders and neck to tighten further, often supplying the "straw" that gave the camel the headache. When the source(s) of the stress subside, the headache will proportionately grow less severe or disappear.

Before closing my discussion about headaches, let me offer one other consideration related to the potential effect on the brain of severe muscle pulling in the head subsystem. Did you ever notice the zig-zag lines that mark the boundaries between the various bones of the skull? Inside these cranial "suture" lines are bundles of connective tissue called Sharpey's fibers. Made of collagen, these fibers help hold the bones of the skull together at the seams created by the suture lines. Many years ago, I learned through experimentation that I could do something with the skull that, at the time, American conventional healthcare said was not possible: manipulate the parietal bones of the skull—probably because of the apparently flexible nature of the Sharpey's fibers in these cranial sutures.

I recalled reading that doctors in Europe took a contrary position. They supposedly believed that these suture line joints were not fused or solid, and were, therefore, somewhat flexible. Encouraged, I decided to experiment with a few patients, and in the process developed a technique for what is best termed "manipulation" of the parietal bones of the skull to see if, as with other moveable joints I manipulated, I saw improvement in a patient experiencing known or suspected symptoms of MSD in the head. To my surprise, I did get some very interesting and positive results. Let me tell you about two of them.

First was the time when a woman at a dinner party complained to me that she could not think clearly, as if she were in a "fog." I palpated her head and found quite a bit of asymmetry. There were what I call "hot" spots—areas of unnatural inflammation on one side, swelling that gave one part of her head a bulging effect and tenderness to the touch on one side. Without massaging her, I placed my palms on her head and applied gentle pressure

in a fashion which, for lack of a more sophisticated term, is best
described as "squeezing." A few minutes later, she reported that her
ability to think clearly had returned, and that she no longer felt as
if she were in a fog. She subsequently came to my office a few times
requesting that I again "squeeze" her head as I had done at the party.
I did so, with the same positive results. On subsequent visits, I also
performed reversal massage in her neck and shoulder areas, for other
symptoms of MSD. Eventually, she no longer complained of having
a foggy mind.

My experience with this woman demonstrated to me that the
suture lines of the parietal bones are somewhat like flexible joints,
and therefore capable of being manipulated. It also showed me how
powerful and extensive the reach of the SLE and MO could be
within the head subsystem and positively supplemented my efforts
to eradicate headaches in a few others.

Another patient—the same one who stopped blistering on
the foot of her normal leg after she ran with a lift in the shoe on
her functional short leg side— had severe tension in her neck and
shoulders. With limited opportunity to visit me because she lived
in a different location, she was willing to endure the post-massage
pain I've mentioned earlier, and so opted to have me perform a
more intense version of reversal massage. About an hour later,
likely as a reaction to the intensity of my massage, she developed
an excruciatingly painful headache that brought her to tears. As I
think back on this situation, though she was less concerned with
labels than relief, this may have qualified as a "migraine." At any
rate, my intuition told me to give her head a "squeeze" or two, so I
did. Within a minute or so, most of her head pain had vanished. She
was a very intelligent and often skeptical woman—very difficult to
impress. The results of my "manipulation" of her head—the almost
instantaneous disappearance of her unbearable head pain—really got
her attention. She shook her head in amazement—but without pain.

I was not amazed, as I had seen this happen before with a few
others on whom I'd put the "squeeze." What this experience did do for
me was to reconfirm how far up the body and how quickly the chain-
reactional pulling from the SLE and MO could reach, how severe the
consequences could be, and how effectively to deal with them.

CHAPTER 15
Diagnosis du Jour: "Fibromyalgia"

In the mid-1990's, I began to hear about what appeared to be a new condition in conventional healthcare lingo, "fibromyalgia." However, the more I heard about it, the more I saw that for the most part it encompassed symptoms of MSD that I had been successfully eliminating for decades. I say, "for the most part," because the literature I found suggested that many people diagnosed with fibromyalgia might also suffer from a number of other conditions. Three of these I have referred to earlier in this book as symptoms of MSD: restless legs syndrome, osteoarthritis, and headaches.

However, the remainder of the other associated conditions were clearly not musculoskeletal in origin: chronic fatigue syndrome, irritable bowel syndrome ("IBS"), lupus, depression, post-traumatic stress disorder, endometriosis, and sleep disorders (including sleep apnea). What's more, over the years I have seen a number of conventional healthcare providers' advertisements that include these unrelated conditions as symptoms of fibromyalgia they claim to be able to eliminate. Given my experience with MSD, I look at fibromyalgia differently than does conventional healthcare. Before I offer my thoughts, I want to summarize what conventional healthcare says about fibromyalgia.

"Fibromyalgia" means "muscle fiber pain." According to conventional healthcare, the muscle fiber pain of fibromyalgia is found in the musculature all over the body, including the tendons and ligaments, as well as at specific locations referred to as "tender points." These tender points are said to be located on the sides and upper reaches of the hips, near the knees, high on the chest, near the shoulders and between the shoulder blades, at the back of the head, on the sides and front of the neck, and on the upper outside portion of the elbows. They're called tender points because these areas hurt when firm pressure is applied. The degree of pain is said to vary with stress and physical activity, among other factors. Conventional healthcare concedes it doesn't know what causes fibromyalgia. It does, however, offer a theoretical explanation for the chronic pain involving a patient's lowered pain threshold and alteration of the brain in such a way as to make it hyper-sensitized to pain.

To treat fibromyalgia chemically, conventional healthcare can offer anti-depressants, analgesics, and/or anti-seizure drugs. Non-chemically, in addition to counseling on how to handle stress, conventional healthcare offers exercise, stretching, and hot or cold packs to help restore muscle balance.

So, what are my thoughts about fibromyalgia? Well, the name is certainly descriptive, as I have maintained all through this book that back and joint pain comes mainly from muscles—and therefore muscle fibers—affected by MO. Otherwise, my opinion is that MSD by any other name should be treated the same. Allow me to explain.

If you've read this far, you may have already noticed that the generalized and "tender point" varieties of fibromyalgia pain look a lot like the "painful-to-the touch" asymmetry and other mild-to-moderate symptoms of MSD I have already mentioned and have consistently maintained are caused by the SLE and MO. You may also recall my general discussion of asymmetries in various areas, including musculature that was not spontaneously painful or painful in use, but was painful to the touch. Think about my description of specific areas in all subsystems that become painful to the touch, such as the upper outsides of the hips, upper chest, and shoulders, and how those painful areas relate to the development of restless legs, osteoarthritis, and headaches. Finally, recall that conventional healthcare tells us that fibromyalgia pain can be worse with physical activity and stress and can respond to stretching and cold packs. Of course it can, because, as I have said all along, this pain is really the development of the less severe symptoms of MSD, caused by the SLE and MO. Moreover, as you understand by now, these milder symptoms of MSD are also predictors of more severe symptoms of MSD to come.

As to what evidence conventional healthcare has to imply statistical association of fibromyalgia and such variant and clearly independent conditions as depression, endometriosis, lupus, and irritable bowel syndrome in its literature and advertisements, I have no idea. At minimum I can say that, as conventional healthcare well knows and must surely have witnessed many times, two or more symptoms with independent causes can exist simultaneously without any cause-and-effect relationship between them. Thus, the implied or claimed cause-and-effect association by conventional healthcare of musculoskeletal and non-musculoskeletal conditions under the name "fibromyalgia" is all the more puzzling, given that conventional healthcare concedes it doesn't know the cause of the musculoskeletal components of fibromyalgia in the first place.

In my practice I diagnosed as symptoms of MSD and eliminated with my massage the generalized areas of pain and "tender points" of many a patient who had previously been given a diagnosis of fibromyalgia by conventional healthcare. Accordingly, to conventional healthcare I respectfully offer my understanding of the cause of and appropriate treatment for the musculoskeletal components of fibromyalgia, and respectfully submit that maybe the legitimacy of the very existence of fibromyalgia as a stand-alone condition should be reconsidered—at the very least, in the context of the musculoskeletal aspects.

CHAPTER 16
Saving the Breast for Last

Undoubtedly you noted my mentioning earlier in this book several examples of asymmetry expressed as differences in one of a woman's breasts compared to the other. If, as you read the chapter on the thoracic subsystem, you were puzzled about why I said nothing about MSD and women's breasts, I apologize. I do, in fact, have something to say about this. Since breast health and appearance is such an important topic, I felt it appropriate to devote a separate chapter addressed to my women readers describing what I've discovered about the relationship between the SLE, MO, and the health and appearance of breasts.

Based on my experiences in my practice dating back over 25 years, I can say that the SLE and MO do indeed create symptoms of MSD that appear in the form of differences in the appearance of the breasts in several ways. Let me tell you what I found and how I found it.

After I became familiar with the symptoms of MSD in the thoracic subsystem outside of the areas in and around the breasts, I began to focus on the asymmetries of the breasts themselves. Apart from noticing the apparently universal "sagging" in the breasts experienced by many—but not exclusively older—women, I also noticed that one breast usually looked different than the other in a number of ways. For example, one would be lower, flatter, or smaller, or would point in a different direction than the other; for example, to the outside as opposed to straight ahead. Also, in some cases, one or both nipples would be recessed or drawn inward instead of protruding—creating difficulty or inability for that woman to breastfeed. My attention also focused on the fact that, particularly in my women patients, I usually found tenderness to the touch in the sternum and underneath one or both breasts. Finally, as I was aware that undergoing a mammogram was a physically uncomfortable and even painful experience for many, if not most, women, I began to wonder how far into the breast the asymmetry of MSD could be found.

Over time, I encountered a few women patients who were open to the idea of exploratory palpation for asymmetries in and around their breasts. Not surprisingly, besides finding their breasts were painful to the touch in many areas, I found asymmetries in the form of knots or other muscle tissue irregularities, taut muscle tissue, and inflammation in the areas around and underlying the fatty part of the breast. As with the others in the thoracic subsystem, these asymmetries and painful areas were usually more pronounced on one side. I suspected that they were also symptoms of MSD created by the SLE and MO. That being the case, I reasoned, I should be able to eliminate these asymmetries through reversal massage.

With the blessing of these women, massage them I did. Though I should not have been surprised by the results, I was nonetheless amazed, especially by the response of the first patient I massaged. In the time it took me to massage the appropriate areas of her thoracic subsystem—less than a half-hour—her upper chest was no longer as receded, and her breasts were noticeably uplifted and thrust forward, resembling more her youth than her age. Also, and even more significantly, she reported that her breathing had improved.

Predictably, the results were the same with each of the other women on whom I massaged the same areas, whether she was in her

30's or her 60's. This again validated my belief that the symptoms of MSD are not a badge of aging, but the result of the effects of the advancement of the SLE due to MO generated, in this case, by the shoulder girdle subsystem. Also, where a patient's nipples were drawn in or recessed, I was likewise able to reverse that aspect of MSD so that the nipples were outward again and were no longer an obstacle to breastfeeding.

So, how and why was I able to uplift the breasts and reverse nipple recession? Again, the "how" was through reversal massage. The simple "why" is that the breasts sagged and the nipples drew inward for the same reason that the buttocks, inner thighs, neck, and chin sag.

The more complex answer is twofold, and goes something like this: A good deal of the breast is composed of fat. However, underlying that fat is muscle tissue that responds to chain-reactional pulling from MO by becoming taut and giving the appearance of being smaller. As with the skin and fat covering the buttocks, inner thighs, neck, and chin, the skin and fat of the breast sag because the muscle underneath is taut and contracted, no longer able to support and help give form to the breast by pushing it upward and outward.

Because of the unique effects of the SLE and MO in the case of the chest, there's another important reason, one that easily can be overlooked. Remember what MO does to the chest in general: it causes it to recede, or cave inward. When it does, the breasts are to a degree drawn back and down, giving the additional appearance of sagging. Thus, between muscle contraction and chest recession, the breasts begin to sag. My reversal massage not only increased the chest volume, but relaxed the muscle fibers underlying the fatty part of the breasts. The entire chest thus increases in volume and is thrust up and out—and the breasts along with it.

And one last thing. Not only does my reversal massage take away the sagging, but there's another, non-cosmetic benefit: at least one patient has confirmed that she no longer experiences pain when lying on her breasts or when undergoing a mammogram.

CHAPTER 17
MSD in Animals?

During the 45 years I spent discovering how the SLE and MO impair the functioning of the musculoskeletal system and how to reverse that impairment, I literally had my hands full focusing on human beings. Even after I retired from active practice many years ago I continued to explore the reversal of MSD, gaining additional insights from some exceptional and interesting patients in the process.

In recent years, though, I began to wonder whether animals, too, have functional short legs or suffer from the effects of muscle overuse. I started observing the gaits of the two animals I have most often encountered in my environment, dogs and cats, wondering if I would find, as I had with humans, anything that might indicate a structural abnormality in either. My curiosity did not disappoint me.

In observing the gait of a number of dogs of different sizes and breeds, I often saw that one leg in a pair moved differently than the other, both in the back and front legs. Whenever the opportunity presented itself, I told the owner that the dog had some problems in that leg. In each case, the understandably surprised owner responded to me by saying, "Yes, I know." In one case, the owner let me palpate the dog. Given what I had seen in the gait of this dog, I was not surprised to find two types of asymmetry that I found in humans: the muscles in the shoulder or hip were much tighter on one side than the other and also had some inflammation. Yet outwardly, the dog exhibited nothing in its behavior or demeanor that I, at least, would recognize as a complaint of pain or discomfort. Recently, with another dog, I was able to take a "dognostic" encounter a bit further.

I walked into the waiting room of a professional office in which the family dog was stretched out on a chair, dozing. This dog, which I had seen in this waiting room before, usually took little more than passing interest in me. On this occasion, though, I called the dog over to me, watching his gait as he approached. I noticed that one of his rear legs moved oddly. When the dog jumped into my lap, I began petting him, and then palpated the hind quarter with the oddly moving leg. As with the other dog, I found uneven muscle tension and inflammation on that leg. Reflexively, I began to massage the tense, inflamed areas for a few minutes. The dog did not flinch or otherwise resist, and in fact appeared to enjoy the rub, like most dogs.

However, when it was time to get up for my appointment, I had a very difficult time getting the dog to leave my lap. When I put him on the floor, he hopped right back up. The look in his eyes said, "I'm not going anywhere. . .don't stop!" The dog's demeanor and reactions suggested that my massage meant far more than just a petting session to him.

I believe that animals that are hurting or sick know when you're trying to help them. My sense was that this dog knew something was wrong in his leg and hip and was feeling better from my massage. Yet as far as I could tell, this dog, like so many others, gave no indication that anything was wrong. Is it that dogs have high pain thresholds, or is it that the pain or discomfort is something they silently suffer until it becomes unbearable? I told the owner, whom I know well, about my experience. He laughed it off.

While I've yet to have the chance to massage or even palpate one, I have observed the same odd gait in cats as well. Of course, I neither am a veterinarian nor possess knowledge about the musculoskeletal system of dogs, cats, or other animals but, as with the patients I saw in my office, I know what I saw and what I discovered when I palpated these animals. It makes me wonder what I might see and palpate in other animals.

I wonder, given the opportunity, what I might find at a greyhound or horse racing track. I wonder if the apparently universal functional short leg, SLE, and MO I found in humans exist in those animals and others and, if so, whether their presence affects the animals' performance in racing, hunting, jumping, tracking, and any number of other physical pursuits such animals follow.

Taking it a bit farther, if I'm right—if animals, too, suffer from MSD—can it be reversed with massage? If a horse had a functional short leg, would it be possible to improve his performance and comfort with an appropriately thicker horseshoe on the functional short leg side? Would it be possible to use reversal massage to reduce the incidence of broken or damaged limbs suffered by so many racehorses? Would it be possible to reduce or eliminate the underlying cause of illness and disability that affect and tragically shorten the lives of our beloved pets with the same techniques that can help us humans to live healthier, more comfortable, and pain-free lives?

I wonder. . .

About the Author

Anthony J. Ippolito was born and raised in Buffalo, New York. After attending Canisius College in Buffalo, he enlisted in the Army Air Force in 1944 and was honorably discharged with the rank of sergeant in 1946. Later that year, he enrolled in Lincoln Chiropractic College in Indianapolis, Indiana. After receiving his Doctor of Chiropractic Degree from Lincoln in 1949, he pursued post-graduate studies in Nutrition and X-ray Interpretation in Radiology at Lincoln before establishing his practice in Buffalo in 1950. After later obtaining licenses to practice chiropractic in Vermont, Kentucky, and Indiana, he relocated his practice to Shelbyville, Indiana in 1959 under the name of Dr. John A. Ramsey. In 1994, after having treated approximately 10,000 patients over 45 years, he retired from active practice. Throughout the1960s he wrote a weekly column on health topics for *The Shelbyville News*. In 1988 he authored an article entitled "Biomechanics" for the October-November issue of *Indy Sports Magazine*. Dr. Ramsey currently lives in Florida.

A Note About the Type

This book is set in Adobe Garamond Pro 12/14. Designed by Claude Garamond (1480-1561), a French publisher and punchcutter who is recognized as the first to make typeface designs available as a service to printers, Garamond is characterized by its elegance, ease of reading, and classic proportions. The Adobe version used to set this book was created by Robert Slimbach in 1989 based on Claude Garamond's original design.